SECOND EDITION

W9-CCH-277

A POCKET GUIDE TO PHYSICAL EXAMINATION AND HISTORY TAKING

SECOND EDITION

A POCKET GUIDE TO PHYSICAL EXAMINATION AND HISTORY TAKING

Barbara Bates, MD

Clinical Professor of Medicine
Medical College of Pennsylvania
Philadelphia, Pennsylvania

Clinical Professor of Nursing
University of Pennsylvania School of Nursing
Philadelphia, Pennsylvania

Lynn S. Bickley, MD

Associate Professor of Medicine
University of Rochester School of Medicine and Dentistry
Rochester, New York

Robert A. Hoekelman, MD

Professor of Pediatrics
University of Rochester School of Medicine and Dentistry

Professor of Nursing
University of Rochester, School of Nursing
Rochester, New York

J. B. Lippincott Company
Philadelphia

Acquisitions Editor: Donna L. Hilton, RN, BSN
Editorial Assistant: Susan M. Keneally
Project Editor: Barbara Ryalls
Manuscript Editor: Mary Norris
Indexer: Katherine Pitcoff
Design Coordinator: Kathy Kelley-Luedtke
Interior Designer: Susan Hess Blaker
Cover Designer: Tom Jackson
Production Manager: Helen Ewan
Production Coordinator: Kathryn Rule
Compositor: Tapsco, Incorporated
Printer/Binder: R. R. Donnelley & Sons Company/Crawfordsville

2nd Edition

6   5   4   3

Bates, Barbara, 1928–
    A pocket guide to physical examination and history taking/
Barbara Bates; with pediatric content by Robert A. Hoekelman.—2nd ed.
        p.   cm.
    Includes bibliographical references and index.
    ISBN 0-397-55057-X (alk. paper)
    1. Physical diagnosis—Handbook, manuals, etc.   2. Medical
history taking—Handbooks, manuals, etc.   I. Hoekelman,
Robert A.   II. Title.
    [DNLM: 1. Medical History Taking—handbooks.
2. Physical Examination—methods—handbooks.
WB 39   B329p   1995]
RC76.B38   1995
6161.07′54—dc20
DNLM/DLC
for Library of Congress   94-16048
                                                                CIP

ACKNOWLEDGMENTS

Mary Norris, editorial designer of the first edition of the *Pocket Guide*, has continued to improve the style and content of this edition. Jennifer Smith created the new line drawings for each of these two editions. We thank them both.

We also appreciate the work of the J. B. Lippincott staff who helped in many additional ways.

C O N T E N T S

Clinical Data

CHAPTER 5

CLINICAL THINKING AND THE PATIENT'S RECORD   209

INTRODUCTION

The *Pocket Guide to Physical Examination and History Taking* is a concise, portable text that

- Outlines the health history
- Provides an illustrated review of the physical examination
- Reminds students of some common findings
- Describes some of the special techniques of assessment that the student may need in specific instances but may not recall in sufficient detail
- Provides succinct aids to interpretation of selected findings

There are several ways to use the *Pocket Guide*:

- To review and thus remember the content of a health history
- To review and rehearse the techniques of examination. This can be done while learning a single section and again while combining the approaches to several body systems or regions into an integrated examination.
- To review some common variations of normal and some selected abnormalities. Observation is more astute when the examiner knows what to look, listen, and feel for.
- To look up special techniques as the need arises. Maneuvers such as everting an eyelid or doing an Allen test are included in the relevant sections of the examination and are initiated by a gray bar. This bar helps readers to use or ignore the special techniques, as they prefer.
- To look up additional information about possible findings, including abnormalities and standards of normal

The *Pocket Guide* is not intended to serve as a primary text from which to learn the skills of taking a history or performing a physical examination. Its detail is insufficient for these purposes. It is intended instead as a mechanism for review and recall and as a convenient, brief, and portable reference.

In this second edition, we have updated the content of the *Pocket Guide*, added some illustrations and special techniques, introduced ten new tables, and expanded several other tables. The purposes and recommended uses of the book remain the same.

CHAPTER 1

THE HEALTH HISTORY

Bates, B. A POCKET GUIDE TO PHYSICAL EXAMINATION AND HISTORY TAKING, SECOND EDITION. © 1995 J.B. Lippincott Company.

Taking a history is usually the first and often the most important part of your interaction with patients. You gather much of the data on which diagnoses are based, you learn about the patients as people and how they have experienced their symptoms and illnesses, and you begin to establish a trusting relationship.

There are several ways to facilitate these goals. Try to provide an environment that is private, quiet, and free of interruption. Seat yourself in a location that is agreeable to the patient, and make sure that he or she is comfortable. Address the patient by name and title, e.g., Mrs. Green, and introduce yourself.

Start the history with open-ended questions: "What brings you to the hospital? . . . Anything else? . . . Tell me about it." Additional ways of encouraging patients to tell their stories include:

Facilitation—posture, actions, or words that communicate interest, such as leaning forward, making eye contact, or saying "Mm-hmmm" or "Go on"

Reflection—repetition of a word or phrase that a patient has used

Clarification—asking what the patient meant by a word or phrase

Empathic responses—recognizing through actions or words the feelings of a patient, such as by offering a tissue or saying "I understand" or "That must have been frightening"

Asking about feelings that a patient has had regarding symptoms, events, or other matters

Confrontation—stating something about the patient's behavior or feelings not expressed verbally or apparently inconsistent with the patient's story

Interpretation—putting into words what you infer about the patient's feelings or about the meaning to the patient of symptoms, events, or other matters

To get specific details, direct questions are often necessary.

- Word them in language understandable to the patient.
- Express them neutrally so as not to bias the patient.
- Ask about one item at a time.
- Proceed from the general to the specific.
- Ask for graded responses rather than a simple yes or no. Multiple-choice questions may also be used.

Some topics may initially be difficult for clinicians to ask about or for patients to discuss, but are very important to include in any history. These include violence and abuse, depression and thoughts of suicide, the use of alcohol and drugs, sexual practices, and sexually transmitted diseases. Review and practice approaches to these topics to be able to explore them effectively.

A COMPREHENSIVE HISTORY OF AN ADULT

DATE of the history

IDENTIFYING DATA: age, sex, race, place of birth, marital status, occupation, and religion

SOURCE OF REFERRAL, if any

SOURCE of the history

RELIABILITY of the history

CHIEF COMPLAINT(S)

PRESENT ILLNESS: a clear, chronological narrative that includes the onset of the problem, the setting in which it developed, its manifestations, and any treatments. The principal symptoms should be described in terms of their seven basic attributes:

- Location
- Quality
- Quantity or severity
- Timing (onset, duration, frequency)
- Setting
- Factors that aggravate or relieve
- Associated manifestations

Note negative data that may have diagnostic significance.

The present illness should also include the patient's understanding of the symptoms and incapacities, his or her responses to them, and the meaning and impact that they have had in the patient's life.

PAST HISTORY

General State of Health
Childhood Illnesses
Adult Illnesses
Psychiatric Illnesses
Accidents and Injuries
Operations
Hospitalizations

CURRENT HEALTH STATUS

Medications, including home remedies, nonprescription drugs, vitamin/mineral supplements, and borrowed medicines, with doses and frequency of use

Allergies

Tobacco, with type, amount, and duration of use

Alcohol, Drugs, and Related Substances

Diet, including usual daily intake of food and beverages

Screening Tests, such as tuberculin test, Pap smears, mammograms, cholesterol level, stools for occult blood

Immunizations, such as tetanus, pertussis, diphtheria, polio, measles, rubella, mumps, influenza, hepatitis B, *Hemophilus influenzae,* type B, and pneumococcal vaccine

Sleep Patterns
Exercise and Leisure
Environmental Hazards, at home, school, and workplace

Safety Measures, such as seat belts

FAMILY HISTORY

- Age and health, or age and cause of death, of parents, siblings, spouse, and children. Data on other relatives may also be useful.
- The occurrence of diabetes, heart disease, hypercholesterolemia, high blood pressure, stroke, kidney disease, tuberculosis, cancer, arthritis, anemia, allergies, asthma, headaches, epilepsy, mental illness, alcoholism, drug addiction, and symptoms like those of the patient

PSYCHOSOCIAL HISTORY

Home Situation and Significant Others, including family and friends

Daily Life over a 24-hour period

Important Experiences, including upbringing, school, military service, work, financial situation, marriage, retirement

Religious Beliefs, if relevant

Outlook on the present and the future

REVIEW OF SYSTEMS

General. Usual weight, recent weight change, fatigue, fever

Skin. Rashes, lumps, sores, itching, dryness, color change, changes in hair or nails

Head. Headaches, head injury

Eyes. Vision, glasses or contact lenses, last eye examination, pain, redness, excessive tearing, double vision, spots, specks, flashing lights, glaucoma, cataracts

Ears. Hearing, tinnitus, vertigo, earaches, infection, discharge

Nose and Sinuses. Frequent colds; nasal stuffiness, discharge, itching; hay fever, nosebleeds, sinus trouble

Mouth and Throat. Condition of teeth and gums, bleeding gums, last dental examination, sore tongue, frequent sore throats, hoarseness

Neck. Lumps in the neck, "swollen glands," goiter, pain or stiffness in the neck

Breasts. Lumps, pain or discomfort, nipple discharge, self-examination

Respiratory. Cough, sputum (color, quantity), hemoptysis, wheezing, asthma, bronchitis, emphysema, pneumonia, tuberculosis, pleurisy; last chest x-ray

Cardiac. Heart trouble, high blood pressure, rheumatic fever, heart murmurs; chest pain or discomfort, palpitations; dyspnea, orthopnea, paroxysmal nocturnal dyspnea, edema; past ECG or other heart tests

Gastrointestinal. Trouble swallowing, heartburn, appetite, nausea, vomiting, regurgitation, vomiting of blood, indigestion. Frequency of bowel movements, color and size of stools, change in bowel habits, rectal bleeding or black tarry stools, hemorrhoids, constipation, diarrhea. Abdominal pain, food intolerance, excessive belching or passing of gas. Jaundice, liver or gallbladder trouble, hepatitis

Urinary. Frequency of urination, polyuria, nocturia, burning or pain on urination, hematuria, urgency, reduced caliber or force of the urinary stream, hesitancy, incontinence; urinary infections, stones

Genital, Male

- Hernias, penile discharge or sores, testicular pain or masses, any sexually transmitted diseases and their treatments, exposure to AIDS, precautions taken against it and other STDs
- Sexual interest, orientation, function, satisfaction, and problems; contraceptive methods

Genital, Female

- Age at menarche; regularity, frequency, and duration of periods; amount of bleeding, bleeding between periods or after intercourse, last menstrual period; dysmenorrhea; premenstrual tension; age at menopause, menopausal symptoms, postmenopausal bleeding
- Discharge, itching, sores, lumps, any sexually transmitted diseases and their treatments, exposure to AIDS, precautions taken against it and other STDs
- Number of pregnancies, number of deliveries, number of abortions (spontaneous and induced); complications of pregnancy; contraceptive methods
- Sexual interest, orientation, function, satisfaction; any problems, including dyspareunia

Peripheral Vascular. Intermittent claudication, leg cramps, varicose veins, clots in the veins

Musculoskeletal. Muscle or joint pains, stiffness, arthritis, gout, backache. If present, describe the location and associated symptoms (swelling, redness, pain, tenderness, stiffness, weakness, limitation of motion or activity).

Neurologic. Fainting, blackouts, seizures, weakness, paralysis, numbness, tingling, tremors or other involuntary movements

Hematologic. Anemia, easy bruising or bleeding, past transfusions and possible reactions

Endocrine. Thyroid trouble, heat or cold intolerance, excessive sweating; diabetes, excessive thirst or hunger, polyuria

Psychiatric. Nervousness, tension, mood including depression; any suicidal ideation; memory

A COMPREHENSIVE PEDIATRIC HISTORY

The child's history follows the same outline as the adult's history, with certain *additions* presented here.

IDENTIFYING DATA: Date and place of birth; nickname; first names of parents (and last name of each, if different)

CHIEF COMPLAINTS. Determine if they are the concerns of the child, the parent(s), a schoolteacher, or some other person.

PRESENT ILLNESS. Determine how each member of the family responds to the child's symptoms, why he or she is concerned, and the secondary gain the child may get from the illness.

PAST HISTORY

Birth History, important when neurologic or developmental problems are present. Get hospital records if necessary.

- Prenatal—maternal health, medications, drug and alcohol use, vaginal bleeding, weight gain, duration of pregnancy
- Natal—nature of labor and delivery, birth weight, Apgar scores at 1 and 5 minutes
- Neonatal—resuscitation efforts, cyanosis, jaundice, infections; nature of bonding

Feeding History, important with under- and overnutrition

- Breast feeding—frequency and duration of feeds, difficulties encountered; timing and method of weaning
- Artificial feeding—type, amount, frequency; vomiting, colic, diarrhea; vitamins, iron, and fluoride supplements; introduction of solid foods
- Eating habits—likes and dislikes, types and amounts of food eaten; parental attitudes and response to feeding problems

Growth and Development History, important with delayed growth, psychomotor and intellectual retardation, and behavioral disturbances

- Physical growth—weight, height, and head circumference at birth and 1, 2, 5, and 10 years; periods of slow or rapid growth
- Developmental milestones—ages child held head up, rolled over, sat, stood, walked, and talked
- Social development—day and night sleeping patterns; toilet training; speech problems; habitual behaviors, discipline problems; school performance; relationships with parents, siblings, and peers

CURRENT HEALTH STATUS

Allergies. Pay particular attention to childhood allergies—eczema, urticaria, perennial allergic rhinitis, asthma, food intolerance, and insect hypersensitivity.

Immunizations. Include dates given and any untoward reactions.

Screening Tests. Include those for vision, hearing, cholesterol, tuberculosis, blood lead, sickle cell disease, and inborn errors of metabolism.

CHAPTER 2

THE PHYSICAL EXAMINATION OF AN ADULT

Bates, B. A POCKET GUIDE TO PHYSICAL EXAMINATION AND HISTORY TAKING, SECOND EDITION. © 1995 J.B. Lippincott Company.

OVERVIEW

For a comprehensive physical examination, use a sequence that maximizes your efficiency and minimizes the patient's effort, yet allows you to be thorough. One such sequence is outlined below, together with symbols that indicate the patient's positions.

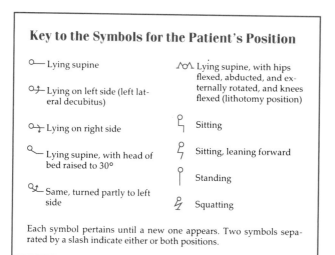

Key to the Symbols for the Patient's Position

○— Lying supine

○⌒ Lying on left side (left lateral decubitus)

○⌒ Lying on right side

○⌒ Lying supine, with head of bed raised to 30°

○⌒ Same, turned partly to left side

∧◇∧ Lying supine, with hips flexed, abducted, and externally rotated, and knees flexed (lithotomy position)

◖ Sitting

◖ Sitting, leaning forward

◖ Standing

◖ Squatting

Each symbol pertains until a new one appears. Two symbols separated by a slash indicate either or both positions.

For the first three sections of this examination, no specific position is necessary.

SEQUENCE OF A COMPREHENSIVE EXAMINATION

General Survey

Mental Status

Skin

Head and Neck, including an initial survey of respiration

Musculoskeletal Examination of the neck and upper back; costovertebral angle tenderness

Posterior Thorax and Lungs

Breast Inspection, Axillae, and Epitrochlear Nodes

Musculoskeletal Examination of the temporomandibular joint and upper extremities, if indicated

Breast Palpation

Anterior Thorax and Lungs

Cardiovascular System

- For finding an elusive apical impulse and for hearing a left-sided S_3 or S_4 and the murmur of mitral stenosis

- For hearing the murmur of aortic regurgitation

Abdomen

Male: Rectum

Female: Genitalia and Rectum

Legs and Feet: peripheral vascular and musculoskeletal examination, and inspection for neurologic findings (position, muscle bulk, involuntary movements)

♀   Varicose Veins

Spine, Legs, and Feet

Male: Genitalia and Hernias

Gait, Romberg test, pronator drift

○—/♀ Neurologic System in detail if indicated:

- Cranial nerves not yet examined

- Motor system: muscle bulk, muscle tone, strength, rapid alternating movements, point-to-point movements

- Sensory system

- Reflexes

The rest of this chapter is devoted to the examination, unit by unit. To facilitate the review or rehearsal of individual body systems or regions, each is described as a whole. The Thorax and Lungs, for example, make up one unit. In practice, however, as shown in the overview above, examination of the breasts and axillae is interposed between the examinations of the posterior thorax and the anterior thorax. Such interpositions or other changes in sequence are indicated by colored shading in the following text.

Special techniques that may not be used often are placed at the end of units and are set off by a gray bar. You may find them there or skip them according to your purpose.

THE GENERAL SURVEY

Examination Techniques	Possible Findings
Check vital signs at outset or later in examination. **Observe** the rest of the following attributes during the interview or examination.	
Apparent State of Health	Robust, acutely or chronically ill, frail
Signs of Distress	Labored breathing, wincing, sweatiness, trembling
Skin Color	Pallor, cyanosis, jaundice
Height and Build	Tall, short, muscular; disproportionately long limbs
Sexual Development	Facial hair, voice changes, breast development
Weight, by appearance or measurement	Emaciated, slender, plump, fat
Posture, Motor Activity, and Gait	Postures to ease breathing or pain; ataxia, a limp, paralysis
Dress, Grooming, and Personal Hygiene	Excessive clothes of hypothyroidism, long sleeves to cover a rash or needle marks
Odors of Body or Breath	Alcohol, odors of diabetic acidosis, uremia, liver failure
Facial Expression	Stare of hyperthyroidism, immobile face of parkinsonism

Examination Techniques	Possible Findings
Speech	Fast speech of hyperthyroidism, hoarseness of myxedema
Vital Signs, including	
• Pulse rate and blood pressure	Tachycardia, hypertension
• Respiratory rate	Tachypnea
• Temperature	Fever, hypothermia

MENTAL STATUS

Observe patient's mental status throughout your interaction. **Test** specific functions if indicated during the interview or physical examination.

APPEARANCE AND BEHAVIOR

Assess the following:

Level of Consciousness. **Observe** patient's alertness and response to verbal and tactile stimuli.	Normal consciousness, lethargy, obtundation, stupor, coma
Posture and Motor Behavior. **Observe** pace, range, character, and appropriateness of movements.	Restlessness, agitation, bizarre postures, immobility, involuntary movements
Dress, Grooming, and Personal Hygiene	Fastidiousness, neglect

Examination Techniques	**Possible Findings**
Facial Expressions during rest and interaction	Anxiety, depression, elation, anger, responses to imaginary people or objects, withdrawal
Manner, Affect, and Relation to Persons and Things	

SPEECH AND LANGUAGE

Note quantity, rate, loudness, clarity, and fluency of speech. If indicated, test for aphasia.	Aphasia, dysphonia, dysarthria, changes with mood disorders

MOOD

Ask about patient's spirits. **Note** nature, intensity, duration, and stability of any abnormal mood. If indicated, **assess** risk of suicide.	Happiness, elation, depression, anxiety, anger, indifference

THOUGHT AND PERCEPTIONS

Thought Processes. **Assess** logic, relevance, organization, and coherence of patient's thought.	Derailments, flight of ideas, incoherence, confabulation, blocking
Thought Content. **Ask** about and **explore** any unusual or unpleasant thoughts.	Obsessions, compulsions, delusions, feelings of unreality
Perceptions. **Ask** about any unusual perceptions, e.g., seeing or hearing things.	Illusions, hallucinations
Insight and Judgment. **Assess** patient's insight into the illness and the level of judgment used in making decisions or plans.	Recognition or denial of the mental cause of symptoms; bizarre, impulsive, or unrealistic judgment

Examination Techniques	**Possible Findings**

COGNITIVE FUNCTIONS

If indicated, **assess:**

Orientation to time, place, and person	Disorientation

Attention

- *Digit span*—the ability to repeat a series of numbers forward and then backward

  Poor performance of digit span, serial 7s, and spelling backward is common in dementia and delirium but has other causes too.

- *Serial 7s*—the ability to subtract 7 repeatedly, starting with 100

- *Spelling backward* of a five-letter word, such as W-O-R-L-D

Remote Memory, e.g., birthdays, anniversaries, social security number, schools, jobs, wars	Impaired in late stages of dementia
Recent memory, e.g., events of the day	Recent memory and new learning ability impaired in dementia, delirium, and amnestic disorders
New learning ability—the ability to repeat three or four words after a few minutes of unrelated activity	

Examination Techniques	Possible Findings

HIGHER COGNITIVE FUNCTIONS

If indicated, **assess:**

Information and Vocabulary. **Note** range and depth of patient's information, complexity of ideas expressed, and vocabulary used. For the fund of information you may also ask names of presidents, other political figures, or large cities.

These attributes reflect intelligence, education, and cultural background. They are limited by mental retardation, but fairly well preserved in early dementia.

Calculating Abilities, such as addition, subtraction, and multiplication

Poor calculation in mental retardation and dementia

Abstract Thinking—the ability to respond abstractly to questions about
- The meaning of *proverbs,* such as "A stitch in time saves nine"
- The *similarities* of beings or things, such as a cat and a mouse or a piano and a violin

Concrete responses common in mental retardation, dementia, and delirium. Responses sometimes bizarre in schizophrenia

Constructional Ability. **Ask** patient

Impaired ability common in dementia and with parietal lobe damage

- To copy figures such as a circle, cross, diamond, and box, and two intersecting pentagons, or

- To draw a clock face with numbers and hands

Examination Techniques	**Possible Findings**

THE SKIN

Examine each region.

SKIN

Inspect and **palpate. Note**

- Color — Cyanosis, jaundice, carotenemia, changes in melanin

- Moisture — Moist, dry, oily

- Temperature — Cool, warm

- Texture — Smooth, rough

- Mobility—the ease with which a fold of skin can be moved — Decreased in edema

- Turgor—the speed with which the fold returns into place — Decreased in dehydration

Note any lesions and their

- Anatomic location — Generalized, localized

- Arrangement — Linear, clustered, dermatomal

- Type — Macule, papule, bulla, tumor

- Color — Red, white, brown, mauve

NAILS

Inspect and **palpate** the fingernails and toenails.

Examination Techniques	**Possible Findings**

Note

- Color   Cyanosis, pallor

- Shape   Clubbing

- Any lesions   Paronychia, onycholysis

HAIR

Inspect and **palpate** the
hair. **Note**

- Quantity   Thin, thick

- Distribution   Patchy or total alopecia

- Texture   Fine, coarse

THE HEAD AND EYES

HEAD

Examine the

- Hair, including quantity,   Coarse and sparse in myx-
  distribution, and texture   edema, fine in hyperthy-
                                 roidism

- Scalp, including lumps or   Pilar cysts, psoriasis
  lesions

- Skull, including size and   Hydrocephalus, skull de-
  contour   pression from trauma

- Face, including symme-   Facial paralysis, emotions
  try and facial expression

- Skin, including color, tex-   Pale, fine, hirsute
  ture, hair distribution,
  and lesions   Acne, skin cancer

Examination Techniques	Possible Findings

EYES

Test visual acuity in each eye.

Diminished acuity

Assess visual fields, if indicated.

Hemianopsia, quadrantic defects

Inspect the

- Position and alignment of eyes

  Exophthalmos, strabismus

- Eyebrows

  Seborrheic dermatitis

- Eyelids

  Sty, chalazion, ectropion, ptosis, xanthelasma

- Lacrimal apparatus

  Swollen lacrimal sac

- Conjunctiva and sclera

  Red eye, jaundice

- Cornea, iris, and lens

  Corneal opacity, cataract

Examine pupils for

- Size, shape, and symmetry

  Miosis, mydriasis, anisocoria

- Reactions to light, and, if these are abnormal—

  Absent in 3rd nerve paralysis

- The near reaction

  Useful in tonic pupils, Argyll Robertson pupils

Assess the extraocular muscles by observing

- The corneal reflections from a midline light

  Muscular imbalance

Examination Techniques	**Possible Findings**
• The six cardinal directions of gaze	Paralytic or nonparalytic strabismus, nystagmus, lid lag

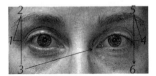

• Convergence	Poor in hyperthyroidism

Inspect the fundi with an ophthalmoscope, including the

• Red reflex	Cataracts, artificial eye
• Optic disc	Papilledema, glaucomatous cupping, optic atrophy

Optic disc   *Fovea*

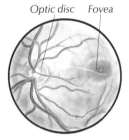

• Arteries, veins, and A–V crossings	Hypertensive changes
• Adjacent retina. **Note** any lesions.	Hemorrhages, exudates, cotton-wool patches, microaneurysms, pigmentation

Examination Techniques	Possible Findings
• Macular area	Macular degeneration
• Anterior structures	Vitreous floaters, cataracts

THE EARS

Examine, on each side:

THE AURICLE

Inspect it.   Keloid, epidermoid cyst

If you suspect otitis,

- Move the auricle up and down, and press on the tragus.   Causes pain in otitis externa

- Press firmly behind the ear.   May be tender in otitis media and mastoiditis

THE EAR CANAL AND EARDRUM

Pull the auricle up, back, and slightly out.

Inspect, through an otoscope speculum,

- The canal   Cerumen, otitis externa

- The eardrum, as illustrated on the next page   Acute otitis media, serous otitis media, tympanosclerosis, perforations

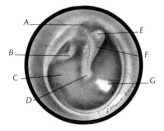

A = Pars flaccida   B = Incus
C= pars tensa   D = Umbo
E= Short process of malleus
F= Handle of malleus
G = Cone of light

(After Hawke M, Keene M, Alberti PW: Clinical Otoscopy: A Text and Colour Atlas. Edinburgh, Churchill Livingstone, 1984)

HEARING

Assess auditory acuity to whispered or spoken voice.

If hearing is diminished, use a 512-Hz tuning fork to

- Test lateralization **(Weber test)**

- Compare air and bone conduction **(Rinne test)**

These tests help to distinguish between sensorineural and conduction hearing loss.

NOSE AND SINUSES

Inspect the external nose.

Inspect, through a speculum, the

Examination Techniques	**Possible Findings**
• Nasal mucosa that covers the septum and turbinates, noting its color and any swelling	Swollen and red in viral rhinitis, swollen and pale in allergic rhinitis; polyps; ulcer from cocaine use
• Nasal septum for position and integrity	Deviation, perforation
Palpate the sinuses for tenderness:	Tender in acute sinusitis
• Frontal	
• Maxillary	

MOUTH AND PHARYNX

Inspect the

• Lips	Cyanosis, pallor, cheilosis
• Oral mucosa	Canker sores
• Gums	Gingivitis, periodontal disease
• Teeth	Dental caries, tooth loss
• Roof of the mouth	Torus palatinus
• Tongue, including	
Papillae	Glossitis
Symmetry	12th cranial nerve paralysis
Any lesions	Cancer of tongue
• Floor of the mouth	Cancer

Examination Techniques	**Possible Findings**

- Pharynx, including

  Color or any exudate | Pharyngitis

  Symmetry of the soft palate as patient says "ah" | 10th cranial nerve paralysis

NECK

Inspect the neck. | Scars, masses, torticollis

Palpate the lymph nodes. | Cervical lymphadenopathy due to inflammation, malignancy

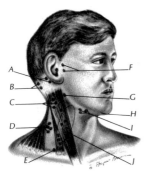

A = Posterior auricular
B = Occipital   C = Superficial cervical   D = Posterior cervical
E = Supraclavicular
F = Preauricular   G = Tonsillar
H = Submental
I = Submandibular   J = Deep cervical chain

Inspect and **palpate** the position of the trachea. | Deviated trachea

Examination Techniques	Possible Findings
Inspect the thyroid gland.	Goiter, nodules
• At rest	
• As patient swallows water	
From behind patient, **palpate** the thyroid gland, including the isthmus and the lateral lobes, as illustrated below.	Goiter, nodules, tenderness of thyroiditis

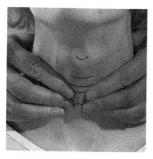

FEELING THE ISTHMUS

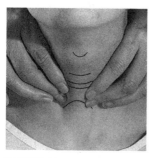

FEELING THE LATERAL LOBES

Examination Techniques	Possible Findings

- At rest

- As patient swallows water

The initial survey of respiration may be done while examining the front of the neck. After feeling the thyroid gland from behind, you may proceed to a musculoskeletal examination of the neck and upper back and a check for costovertebral angle tenderness.

S P E C I A L   T E C H N I Q U E S

EVERSION OF THE UPPER EYELID. The patient should relax and look down.

Grasp eyelashes of upper lid and pull them gently down and forward.

Place an applicator stick or the edge of a tongue blade horizontally on upper lid at least 1 cm above lid margin, and push it down on eyelid, thus everting lid.

Hold lashes of upper lid against eyebrow while you inspect the palpebral conjunctiva.

When finished, pull eyelashes gently forward, and ask patient to look up.

Eversion of lid reveals foreign bodies and lesions of the palpebral conjunctiva of upper lid.

Examination Techniques	Possible Findings

℔   FOR NASOLACRIMAL DUCT OBSTRUCTION. As patient looks up, press on lower lid near medial canthus and just inside rim of bony orbit. Look for fluid coming out of puncta into eye.

Regurgitation of mucopurulent fluid from puncta suggests obstructed duct and may identify cause of excessive tearing. Avoid this test if area is inflamed and tender.

℔/℔   TRANSILLUMINATION OF THE FRONTAL AND MAXILLARY SINUSES. In a fully darkened room, shine a bright narrow light

A local red glow in the forehead or in the roof of the mouth suggests that the frontal or maxillary sinus, respectively, is air filled. Absence of a glow suggests a thickened mucosa or secretions.

- Upward under each brow. Shield light with your hand and observe forehead.

- Downward from just below the inner aspect of each eye. Patient's head should be tilted back, with mouth open. Observe roof of mouth.

THE THORAX AND LUNGS

℔   SURVEY

Inspect the thorax and its respiratory movements. **Note**

- Rate, rhythm, depth, and effort of breathing

  Tachypnea, hyperpnea, Cheyne–Stokes breathing

- Inspiratory retraction of the supraclaviclar areas

  Occurs in COPD, asthma, upper airway obstruction

Examination Techniques	Possible Findings
• Inspiratory contraction of the sternomastoids	Indicates severe breathing difficulty
Observe shape of patient's chest.	Normal or barrel chest
Listen to patient's breathing for	
• Stridor	Stridor in upper airway obstruction
• Wheezes	Wheezes in obstructive lung disease

THE POSTERIOR CHEST

Inspect the chest for

• Deformities or asymmetry	Kyphoscoliosis
• Abnormal inspiratory retraction of the interspaces	Retraction in airway obstruction
• Impairment or unilateral lag in respiratory movement	Disease of the underlying lung or pleura

Palpate the chest for

• Tender areas	Fractured ribs
• Assessment of visible abnormalities	Masses, sinus tracts
• Respiratory expansion	Impairment, one or both sides
• Tactile fremitus	Local or generalized decrease or increase

Examination Techniques	Possible Findings

Percuss the chest in the areas illustrated, comparing one side with the other at each level.

Dullness occurs when fluid or solid tissue replaces normally air-filled lung. Hyperresonance often accompanies emphysema or pneumothorax.

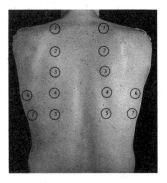

Identify level of diaphragmatic dullness on each side and **estimate** diaphragmatic excursion.

Pleural effusion or a paralyzed diaphragm raises level of dullness.

Listen to chest with stethoscope in areas shown above, again comparing sides.

• Evaluate the breath sounds.

Vesicular, bronchovesicular, or bronchial breath sounds; decreased breath sounds from decreased air flow

• Note any adventitious (added) sounds.

Crackles (fine and coarse) and continuous sounds (wheezes and rhonchi)

Observe their qualities, place in the respiratory cycle, and location on the chest

Examination Techniques   **Possible Findings**

wall. Do they clear with
deep breathing or coughing?

Assess transmitted voice
sounds if you have heard
bronchial breath sounds in
abnormal places. Ask pa-
tient to

- Say "99" and "ee"   Bronchophony, egophony,
                             and whispered pectoriloquy

- Whisper "99" or "1, 2, 3"

While the patient is still sitting, you may inspect the
breasts and examine the axillary and epitrochlear
lymph nodes. If indicated, also examine the temporomandibular joint and the musculoskeletal system of
the upper extremities.

o— THE ANTERIOR CHEST

Inspect the chest for

- Deformities or asym-   Pectus excavatum
  metry

- Intercostal retraction   From obstructed airways

- Impaired or lagging re-   From disease of the underly-
  spiratory movement   ing lung or pleura

Palpate the chest for

- Tender areas   Tender pectoral muscles,
                             costochondritis

Examination Techniques	Possible Findings
• Assessment of visible abnormalities	Flail chest
• Respiratory expansion	
• Tactile fremitus	
Percuss the chest in the areas illustrated.	Normal cardiac dullness may disappear in emphysema.

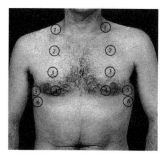

Listen to chest with stethoscope. **Note**

• Breath sounds

• Adventitious sounds

• If indicated, transmitted voice sounds

| **Examination Techniques** | **Possible Findings** |

S P E C I A L   T E C H N I Q U E S

ASSESSMENT OF
PULMONARY FUNCTION.
If appropriate, walk with
patient down the hall or up
a flight of stairs. Observe
rate, effort, and sound of
breathing, and inquire about
symptoms.

FORCED EXPIRATORY
TIME. Ask patient to take a
deep breath in and then
breathe out as quickly and
completely as possible, with
mouth open. Listen over trachea with diaphragm of
stethoscope and time audible expiration. Try to get
three consistent readings, al-
lowing rests as needed.

If the patient understands
and cooperates well, a
forced expiratory time of 6
or more seconds strongly
suggests obstructive pulmonary disease.

IDENTIFICATION OF
A FRACTURED RIB. Point
tenderness of a rib suggests
fracture but may be due to
soft-tissue injury. With one
hand on patient's sternum
and the other on the thoracic
spine, squeeze patient's
chest. Does this anteroposterior compression cause
pain? If so, where?

An increase in local rib pain,
distant from your hands,
suggests rib fracture rather
than just soft-tissue injury.

Examination Techniques	**Possible Findings**

THE BREASTS AND AXILLAE

♀   FEMALE BREASTS

Inspect the breasts for

• Size and symmetry	Development, asymmetry
• Contour	Flattening, dimpling
• Appearance of the skin	Edema (peau d'orange) in breast cancer

Inspect the nipples.

• Compare their size, shape, and direction of pointing	Inversion, retraction, deviation
• Note any rashes, ulcerations, or discharge.	Paget's disease of the nipple, galactorrhea

Continue your inspection as patient

• Raises both arms above her head	Dimpling and abnormalities of contour
• Presses her hands against her hips	

○—   **Palpate** the breasts for

• Consistency	Physiologic nodularity
• Tenderness	Infection, premenstrual tenderness

Examination Techniques	**Possible Findings**
• Nodules. If present, **note** their	Cyst, fibroadenoma, cancer
Location	
Size	
Shape	
Consistency	
Delimitation	
Tenderness	
Mobility	
Palpate each nipple.	Thickening in cancer
Compress the areola in a spokelike pattern around the nipple if patient has reported spontaneous nipple discharge. **Watch** for discharge.	Type and source of discharge may thereby be identified.

♂ MALE BREASTS

Inspect the nipple and areola.	Gynecomastia, cancer
Palpate the areola and adjacent area.	Gynecomastia, cancer, fat

♀ AXILLAE

Inspect for rashes, infection, and pigmentation.	Hidradenitis suppurativa, acanthosis nigricans
Palpate the central axillary nodes.	Lymphadenopathy

Examination Techniques	**Possible Findings**

If indicated, **palpate** the other axillary nodes:

- Pectoral group

- Lateral group

- Subscapular group

THE CARDIOVASCULAR SYSTEM

⚲ THE ARTERIAL PULSE

RADIAL ARTERY

Palpate the radial pulse. **Note**

- Heart rate	Tachycardia, bradycardia
- Rhythm. If this is irregular, listen to the heart.	Premature contractions, atrial fibrillation

CAROTID ARTERY

Palpate the carotid artery pulse. **Note**

- Amplitude	Increased, decreased
- Any variations in amplitude	Pulsus alternans
- Contour	Rapid upstroke and fall in aortic regurgitation
- Any thrills	

Listen with a stethoscope for a bruit or a murmur transmitted from the heart. — Bruit and possible thrill in carotid obstruction; transmitted murmur of aortic stenosis

Examination Techniques	**Possible Findings**

BLOOD PRESSURE

Estimate systolic blood pressure by palpation and **add** 30 mm Hg. Use this sum as the target for further cuff inflations.

This step helps you to detect an auscultatory gap.

Measure blood pressure with a sphygmomanometer.

If indicated, **check** it

Orthostatic (postural) hypotension

JUGULAR VEINS

Identify the jugular venous pulsations and their highest point in the neck. Adjust angle of bed as necessary.

Measure jugular venous pressure—the vertical distance between this highest point and the sternal angle, normally less than 3–4 cm.

Elevated venous pressure in right-sided heart failure

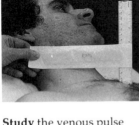

Study the venous pulse waves.

Absent *a* waves in atrial fibrillation

| **Examination Techniques** | **Possible Findings** |

THE HEART

Inspect and **palpate** the anterior chest for pulsations.

Identify the apical impulse. Turn patient to left as necessary. **Note**

- Location of impulse

    Displaced to left in pregnancy.

- Diameter

    Increased diameter, amplitude, and duration in left ventricular enlargement

- Amplitude

- Duration

Feel for a right ventricular impulse in left parasternal and epigastric areas.

Prominent impulses suggest right ventricular enlargement.

Palpate left and right second interspaces close to sternum. **Note** any thrills in these areas.

Pulsations of great vessels; accentuated S_2; thrills of aortic or pulmonic stenosis

Listen to heart with stethoscope. Use its diaphragm in all areas illustrated on p. 42 and its bell at the apex and the lower left sternal border.

Examination Techniques   Possible Findings

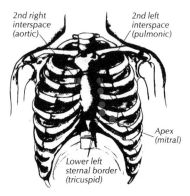

2nd right interspace (aortic)

2nd left interspace (pulmonic)

Apex (mitral)

Lower left sternal border (tricuspid)

Listen at each area:

- To S_1

- To S_2. Is splitting normal in left 2nd and 3rd interspaces? — Physiologic (inspiratory) or pathologic (expiratory) splitting

- For extra sounds in systole — Systolic clicks

- For extra sounds in diastole — S_3, S_4

- For systolic murmurs — Midsystolic, pansystolic, late systolic murmurs

- For diastolic murmurs — Early, mid-, or late diastolic murmurs

Identify, if murmurs are present, their

- Timing in the cardiac cycle (systole, diastole)

Examination Techniques	Possible Findings
• Shape	Plateau, crescendo, decrescendo
• Location of maximal intensity	
• Radiation	
• Intensity on a 6-point scale	
• Pitch	High, medium, low
• Quality	Blowing, harsh, musical, rumbling

Listen at the apex with patient turned toward left side.

Left-sided S_3, S_4, and murmur of mitral stenosis

Listen down left sternal border to the apex as patient sits, leaning forward, with breath held in exhalation.

Murmur of aortic regurgitation

SPECIAL TECHNIQUES

PULSUS ALTERNANS. Feel pulse for alternation in amplitude. Lower pressure of blood pressure cuff slowly to systolic level while you listen with stethoscope over brachial artery.

Alternating amplitude of pulse or sudden doubling of Korotkoff sounds indicates a pulsus alternans—a sign of left ventricular failure.

PARADOXICAL PULSE. Lower pressure of blood pressure cuff slowly and note two pressure lev-

A difference greater than 10 mm Hg signifies a paradoxical pulse. Consider obstructive lung disease, pericardial

Examination Techniques	Possible Findings

els: (1) where Korotkoff sounds are first heard, and (2) where they first persist through the respiratory cycle. These levels are normally not more than 3–4 mm Hg apart.

tamponade, or constrictive pericarditis.

VALSALVA MANEUVER. Ask patient to strain down. In suspected *mitral valve prolapse (MVP)*, listen to the timing of click and murmur.

The systolic click of MVP becomes earlier, and the murmur lengthens.

To distinguish *aortic stenosis (AS)* from *hypertrophic cardiomyopathy (HC)*, listen to the intensity of the murmur.

In AS, the murmur decreases; in HC, it often increases.

SQUATTING AND STANDING. In suspected *MVP*, listen for the click and murmur in both positions.

Squatting delays the click and murmur. Standing reverses the changes.

Try to distinguish *AS* from *HC* by listening to the murmur in both positions.

Squatting increases murmur of AS and decreases murmur of HC. Standing reverses the changes.

THE ABDOMEN

Inspect the abdomen, including

• Skin

Scars, striae, veins

• Umbilicus

Hernia, inflammation

Examination Techniques	Possible Findings
• Contours for shape, symmetry, enlarged organs or masses	Bulging flanks, suprapubic bulge, large liver or spleen, tumors
• Any peristaltic waves	GI obstruction
• Any pulsations	Increased in aortic aneurysm

Auscultate the abdomen, if indicated clinically, for

• Bowel sounds	Increased or decreased motility
• Bruits	Bruit of renal artery stenosis

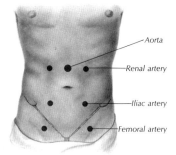

Aorta
Renal artery
Iliac artery
Femoral artery

• Friction rubs	Liver tumor, splenic infarct
Percuss the abdomen for proportions and patterns of tympany and dullness	Ascites, GI obstruction, pregnant uterus, ovarian tumor

Palpate all quadrants of the abdomen

• Lightly for guarding and tenderness	Peritoneal inflammation

Examination Techniques	**Possible Findings**

- Deeply for masses or tenderness

Tumors, a distended viscus

THE LIVER

Percuss span of liver dullness in midclavicular line (MCL).

Hepatomegaly

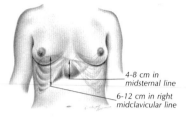

4-8 cm in
midsternal line

6-12 cm in right
midclavicular line

Feel the liver edge, if possible, as patient breathes in.

Firm edge of cirrhosis

Measure its distance from the costal margin in the MCL.

Increased in hepatomegaly

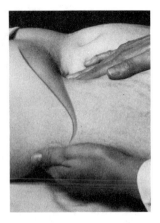

Examination Techniques	**Possible Findings**

Note any tenderness or masses.

Tender liver of hepatitis or congestive heart failure; tumor mass

THE SPLEEN

Percuss across left lower anterior chest, noting change from tympany to dullness.

Check for a splenic percussion sign.

Try to **feel** spleen with the patient:

Splenomegaly

• Supine

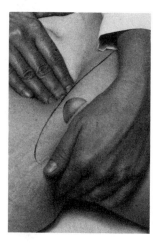

○⌐   • Lying on the right side

Examination Techniques   **Possible Findings**

○— **THE KIDNEYS**

Try to **palpate** each kidney.

Enlargement from cysts, cancer, hydronephrosis

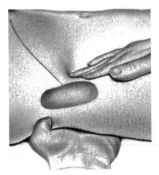

Check for costovertebral angle tenderness.

Tender in kidney infection

○— **THE AORTA**

Palpate the aorta's pulsations and, in older people, **estimate** its width.

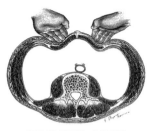   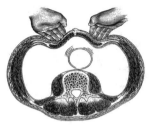

ABDOMINAL AORTA   **AORTIC ANEURYSM**

Examination Techniques	Possible Findings

SPECIAL TECHNIQUES

REBOUND TENDER-NESS. Press slowly on a tender area, then quickly withdraw your hand. Greater pain on withdrawal is rebound tenderness.

Rebound tenderness suggests peritoneal inflammation.

SHIFTING DULL-NESS IN ASCITES. Map areas of tympany and dullness with patient supine and lying on side.

Ascitic fluid usually shifts to dependent side, changing the margin of dullness.

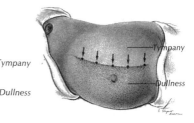

FLUID WAVE IN ASCITES. Ask patient or an assistant to press edges of both hands into midline of abdomen. Tap one side, and feel for a wave transmitted to the other side.

A palpable wave suggests but does not prove ascites.

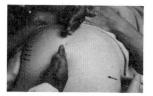

Examination Techniques	Possible Findings

o— HOOKING TECH-NIQUE FOR PALPATING LIVER. Stand to right of patient's chest and place both hands side by side with fingers below lower border of liver dullness. Press in and up and try to feel liver as patient breathes in.

A liver that is not palpable by the usual method is sometimes felt this way.

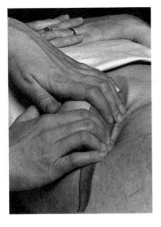

o— MURPHY'S SIGN FOR ACUTE CHOLECYSTITIS. Hook your thumb under right costal margin at edge of rectus muscle, and ask patient to take a deep breath.

Sharp tenderness and a sudden stop in inspiratory effort constitutes a positive sign.

Examination Techniques	**Possible Findings**

o— BALLOTTEMENT. To find an organ or mass in an ascitic abdomen, try to ballotte it. Place your stiffened and straightened fingers on the abdomen, briefly jab them toward the structure, and try to touch its surface.

Your hand, quickly displacing the fluid, stops abruptly as it touches the solid surface.

o— ASSESSING POSSIBLE APPENDICITIS, the basic approach:

In classic appendicitis:

"Where did the pain begin?"   Near the umbilicus

"Where is it now?"   Right lower quadrant

Ask patient to cough. "Where does it hurt?"   Right lower quadrant

Search for local tenderness.   RLQ tenderness

Feel for muscular rigidity.   RLQ rigidity

Perform a rectal exam and, in women, a pelvic exam.   Possibly local tenderness, especially if appendix is retrocecal

Examination Techniques   **Possible Findings**

MALE GENITALIA

This examination is usually deferred until the patient is standing.

Wear gloves.

 THE PENIS

Inspect the

• Development of the penis and the skin and hair at its base	Sexual maturation, lice
• Prepuce	Phimosis
• Glans	Balanitis, chancre, herpes, warts, cancer
• Urethral meatus	Hypospadias, discharge of urethritis

Palpate

• Any visible lesions	Chancre, cancer
• The shaft	Urethral stricture or cancer

THE SCROTUM AND ITS CONTENTS

Inspect

• Contours of scrotum	Hernia, hydrocele, cryptorchidism
• Skin of scrotum	Rashes

Examination Techniques	**Possible Findings**

Palpate each

- Testis, noting any

Lumps	Cancer
Tenderness	Orchitis, torsion

- Epididymis | Epididymitis, cyst

- Spermatic cord and adjacent areas | Varicocele

HERNIAS

Inspect inguinal and femoral areas as patient strains down.

Inguinal and femoral hernias

Palpate external inguinal ring through scrotal skin, and ask patient to strain down.

Indirect and direct inguinal hernias

S P E C I A L   T E C H N I Q U E

TRANSILLUMINATION OF A SCROTAL MASS. Darken room, and shine beam of a good flashlight from behind scrotum through mass. Note whether mass lights up with a red glow.

Fluid-filled masses such as cysts light up; those containing blood or solid tissue do not.

Examination Techniques   **Possible Findings**

ANUS, RECTUM, AND PROSTATE—MALE

Inspect the

- Sacrococcygeal area

  Pilonidal cyst or sinus

- Perianal area

  Hemorrhoids, warts, herpes, chancre, cancer

Palpate the anal canal and rectum with a lubricated and gloved finger. Feel the

- Walls of the rectum

  Cancer of the rectum, polyps

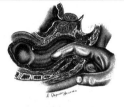

- Prostate gland, as shown below

  Benign hyperplasia, cancer, acute prostatitis

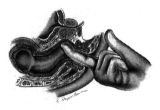

Try to **feel** above the prostate for irregularities or tenderness, if indicated.

Rectal shelf of peritoneal metastases; tenderness of inflammation

| **Examination Techniques** | **Possible Findings** |

FEMALE GENITALIA, ANUS, AND RECTUM

Wear gloves.

EXTERNAL GENITALIA

o— **Observe** pubic hair to assess sexual maturity.

Normal or delayed puberty

ᴧᴧ **Inspect** the

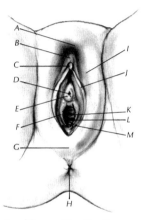

A = Mons pubis   B = Prepuce
C= Clitoris   D = Urethral orifice
E= Opening of Skene's gland
F= Vestibule   G = Perineum
H= Anus   I = Labium majus
J= Labium minus   K = Hymen
L= Vagina   M = Opening of
Bartholin's gland

• Labia	Inflammation
• Clitoris	Enlarged in masculinization
• Urethral orifice	Urethral caruncle
• Introitus	Imperforate hymen

Examination Techniques	**Possible Findings**
Palpate for enlargement or tenderness of Bartholin's glands.	Bartholin's gland infection
Milk the urethra for discharge, if indicated.	Discharge of urethritis

INTERNAL EXAMINATION

Locate the cervix with a gloved and water-lubricated index finger.	
Assess support of vaginal outlet by asking patient to strain down.	Cystocele, cystourethrocele, rectocele
Enlarge the introitus by pressing its posterior margin downward.	
Insert a water-lubricated speculum of suitable size, starting with speculum held obliquely.	

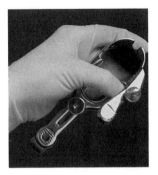

ENTRY ANGLE

Examination Techniques	Possible Findings

Rotate speculum, open it and inspect cervix.

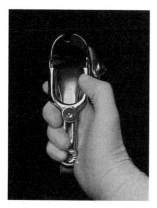

ANGLE AT FULL INSERTION

Observe

- Position

  Cervix faces forward if uterus is retroverted.

- Color

  Purplish in pregnancy

- Epithelial surface

  Squamous and columnar epithelium

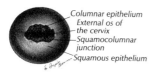

Columnar epithelium
External os of the cervix
Squamocolumnar junction
Squamous epithelium

- Any discharge or bleed-ing

  Discharge from os in muco-purulent cervicitis

- Any ulcers, nodules, or masses

  Herpes, polyp, cancer

Examination Techniques	Possible Findings
Obtain specimens for cytology (Pap smears) with	Early cancer before it is clinically evident
• An endocervical swab and a spatula to scrape the ectocervix	
• Or, if the woman is not pregnant, a cervical brush for a combined specimen	
Inspect the vaginal mucosa as you withdraw the speculum.	Bluish color and deep rugae in pregnancy; vaginal cancer
Palpate the cervix and fornices.	Pain on moving cervix in pelvic inflammatory disease
Palpate, by means of a bimanual examination,	
• The uterus	Pregnancy, myomas; soft isthmus in early pregnancy
• Right and left adnexa	Ovarian masses, salpingitis, tubal pregnancy
Assess strength of pelvic muscles. With your vaginal fingers clear of the cervix, ask patient to tighten her muscles around your fingers as hard and long as she can.	A firm squeeze that compresses your fingers, moves them up and inward, and lasts more than 3 seconds is full strength.
Perform a rectovaginal examination.	Retroverted uterus

Examination Techniques	Possible Findings

ANUS AND RECTUM

♂/♀ **Inspect** the anus.

Hemorrhoids

Palpate the anal canal and rectum.

Rectal cancer, normal uterine cervix or tampon (felt through rectal wall)

SPECIAL TECHNIQUE

HERNIAS. Ask the patient to strain down, as you palpate for a bulge in

- The femoral canal

  Femoral hernia

- The labia majora up to just lateral to the pubic tubercle

  Indirect inguinal hernia

THE PERIPHERAL VASCULAR SYSTEM

Inspection of the limbs may also include findings relevant to the musculoskeletal and nervous systems.

ARMS
Inspect for

- Size and symmetry, any swelling

  Lymphedema, venous obstruction

- Venous pattern

  Venous obstruction

- Color and texture of skin and nails

  Raynaud's disease

Examination Techniques	Possible Findings

Palpate the pulses:

- Radial

Lost in thromboangiitis obliterans or acute arterial occlusion

- Brachial

Feel for the epitrochlear nodes.

Lymphadenopathy

○— **LEGS**

Inspect for

- Size and symmetry, any swelling

Venous insufficiency, lymphedema

- Venous pattern

Varicose veins

- Color and texture of skin

Pallor, rubor, cyanosis

- Hair distribution

Loss in arterial insufficiency

Check for pitting edema.

Peripheral or systemic causes of edema

Palpate the pulses:

Loss of pulses in acute arterial occlusion and arteriosclerosis obliterans

- Femoral

- Popliteal

- Dorsalis pedis

- Posterior tibial

Palpate the inguinal lymph nodes:

Lymphadenopathy

Examination Techniques	Possible Findings

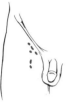

- Horizontal group

- Vertical group

Ask patient to stand, and reinspect the venous pattern.

Varicose veins

SPECIAL TECHNIQUES

EVALUATING ARTERIAL SUPPLY TO HAND. Feel ulnar pulse, if possible. Perform an **Allen test.** Ask patient to make a tight fist, palm up. Occlude both radial and ulnar arteries with your thumbs. Ask patient to open hand into a relaxed, slightly flexed position. Release your pressure over one artery. Palm should flush within about 3–5 seconds. Repeat, releasing other artery.

Persisting pallor of palm indicates occlusion of the released artery or its distal branches.

POSTURAL COLOR CHANGES OF CHRONIC ARTERIAL INSUFFICIENCY. Raise both legs to about 60° for about a minute. Then ask

Marked pallor of feet on elevation, delayed color return and venous filling, and rubor of dependent feet suggest arterial insufficiency.

Examination Techniques	Possible Findings

patient to sit up with legs dangling down. Note time required for (1) return of pinkness, normally about 10 seconds or less, and (2) filling of veins on feet and ankles, normally about 15 seconds. Watch for development of any unusual rubor.

THE MUSCULOSKELETAL SYSTEM

Screening

Inspect the joints and surrounding tissues as you examine the various parts of the body.

Observe

- Ease and range of motion

- Any signs of inflammation in or around joints

- Condition of surrounding tissues

- Any musculoskeletal deformities, including abnormal curvatures of the spine

Assess the spine, especially during adolescence.

Asymptomatic scoliosis often becomes evident in adolescence.

Examination Techniques	Possible Findings

Outlined below is an examination appropriate to a patient with joint symptoms.

HEAD AND NECK

Palpate the temporomandibular joint as patient opens and closes mouth.	Swelling, tenderness, and decreased motion in arthritis
Inspect the neck for deformities.	Torticollis; immobility in ankylosing spondylitis
Palpate the cervical spine and muscles from behind patient.	Local tenderness

Test the range of neck motion in

- Flexion

- Extension

- Rotation

- Lateral bending

HANDS AND WRISTS

Ask patient to

• Make a fist with each hand	Consider functional significance and diagnostic meaning of limited motion.

- Straighten fingers

- Flex and extend wrists

- Turn hands (with palms down) laterally and medially (lateral and medial deviation)

Examination Techniques	**Possible Findings**
Inspect hands and wrists.	Deformities, swelling, muscular atrophy

Palpate

• Distal and proximal interphalangeal joints	Proximal joint swelling in rheumatoid arthritis; distal nodules of osteoarthritis (Heberden's nodes)

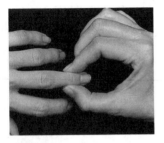

• Metacarpophalangeal joints	Swelling in rheumatoid arthritis

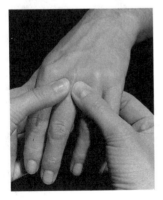

Examination Techniques	Possible Findings
• Wrist joints	Wrist swelling in rheumatoid arthritis and in gonococcal infection of the joint or extensor tendon sheaths

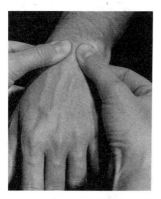

ELBOWS

Ask patient to

• Bend and straighten elbows

• Turn palms up and down (supination and pronation of forearms)

Inspect and **palpate** the elbows, including the

• Olecranon process	Olecranon bursitis
• Grooves overlying the elbow joint	Tenderness in arthritis
• Medial and lateral epicondyles	Tender in epicondylitis
• Extensor surface of the ulna	Rheumatoid nodules

Examination Techniques   **Possible Findings**

SHOULDERS

Ask patient to

- Raise both arms verti-
  cally

  Consider functional significance to patient when these
  or other movements are
  limited.

- Place both hands behind
  neck with elbows out
  (abduction and external
  rotation)

- Place both hands behind
  small of back (internal
  rotation)

Inspect shoulders and
shoulder girdles from front
and back.

Muscular atrophy

Palpate for tenderness, including areas illustrated.

Rotator cuff tendinitis is the
most common cause of sub-
acromial tenderness (B).

Tenderness at A in bicipital
tendinitis

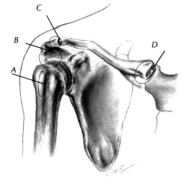

A = Bicipital groove
B = Subacromial area
C = Acromioclavicular joint
D = Sternoclavicular joint

Examination Techniques	**Possible Findings**

○— ANKLES AND FEET

Inspect ankles and feet.

Hallux valgus, corns, calluses

Palpate ankle joints.

Tender joint in arthritis; tender ligaments in a sprain

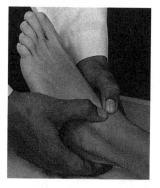

Feel along the Achilles tendons.

Rheumatoid nodules

Squeeze each forefoot, thus compressing the metatarsophalangeal joints; then **pal-**

Tenderness in arthritis and other conditions

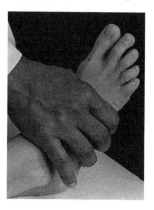

Examination Techniques   Possible Findings

pate each joint between
your thumb and finger.

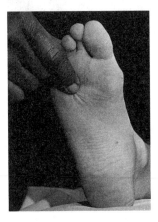

Assess range of motion.

- Dorsiflex and plantar flex
  foot at ankle (tibiotalar
  joint).

- Stabilize ankle with one
  hand and invert and
  evert heel (subtalar joint).

An arthritic joint often hurts
when moved in any direc-
tion. A sprain hurts chiefly
when the injured ligament is
stretched.

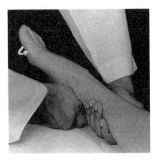

INVERSION

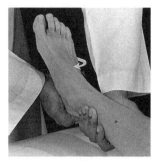

EVERSION

- Stabilize heel and invert and evert forefoot (transverse tarsal joint).

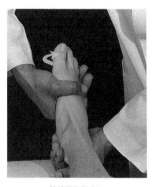

INVERSION

Examination Techniques   **Possible Findings**

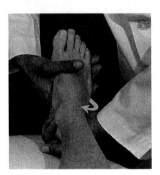

EVERSION

- Flex toes at metatarso-
  phalangeal joints.

KNEES AND HIPS

Inspect and **palpate** each   Bowlegs, knock-knees
knee, including the

- Area of the suprapatellar   Swelling above and beside
  pouch   patella suggests excessive
                                     fluid in the suprapatellar
                                     pouch and in the knee joint.
- Hollow on each side of
  the patella

- Patella   Swelling of prepatellar
                                     bursitis

Assess the patellofemoral
compartment.

- Pressing on patella, move   Pain and crepitus on these
  it against underlying   two maneuvers, along with
  femur.   a history of knee pain, sug-
                                     gest a patellofemoral
                                     disorder.

- Push patella distally and
  ask patient to tighten
  knee against table.

Examination Techniques	**Possible Findings**

With patient's knee flexed to 90°, **palpate** the tibiofemoral joint.

Tenderness of an injured prepatellar fat pad or injured meniscus

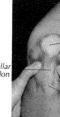

Patellar tendon

Patella
Lateral epicondyle
Lateral collateral ligament
Tibia
Tibial tuberosity

Check range of motion, including

• Flexion at hip and knee

Flexion of opposite leg suggests a flexion deformity of that hip.

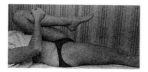

• Rotation at hip, both external (shown below) and internal

Restricted in arthritis

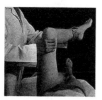

Examination Techniques   **Possible Findings**

- Abduction at hip   Restricted in arthritis

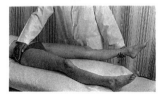

Palpate the following areas
when indicated by pain or is
limited motion:

- The *hip joint* and *iliopec-*   Tender in synovitis, bursitis,
  tineal bursa, lateral to the   iliopsoas abscess
  femoral pulse

- The *trochanteric*   Tender in bursitis
  bursa, on the greater tro-
  chanter of the femur

- The *ischial bursa*, super-   Tender in bursitis
  ficial to the ischial tuber-
  osity

    Observe any deform-   Popliteal swelling of a
ities of knees or feet when   Baker's cyst, flat feet
patient stands.

THE SPINE

Inspect spine from side and   Kyphosis, scoliosis, lordosis,
back, noting any abnormal   gibbus, list
curvatures. Look for any
asymmetries of shoulders,
iliac crests, or buttocks.   Pelvic tilt

| **Examination Techniques** | **Possible Findings** |

Check range of motion in

- Flexion. Watch for normal flattening of lumbar curve.

  Persisting lumbar concavity and decreased range of motion due to muscle spasm, disc disease, or ankylosing spondylitis

- Lateral bending

- Extension

- Rotation

Palpate for tenderness of the

Tenderness from disc disease, muscle spasm, compression fracture, and other conditions

- Spinous processes

- Paravertebral muscles

S P E C I A L   T E C H N I Q U E S

○— STRAIGHT LEG RAISING. Raise patient's straightened leg until pain occurs. Then dorsiflex foot.

Sharp pain down back of leg suggests tension on or compression of a nerve root. Dorsiflexion increases pain.

⌐ PHALEN'S TEST FOR CARPAL TUNNEL SYNDROME. Hold patient's wrists in acute flexion, or ask patient to press backs of both hands together to form right angles as illustrated on p. 74. Either position should be held for 60 seconds.

Numbness or tingling over distribution of median nerve is a positive sign, suggesting carpal tunnel syndrome.

Examination Techniques   Possible Findings

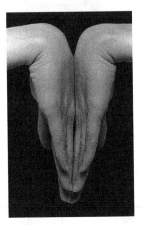

PHALEN'S TEST

TINEL'S SIGN FOR CARPAL TUNNEL SYNDROME. Percuss lightly over median nerve at wrist.

Tingling or an electric sensation in distribution of median nerve is a positive sign.

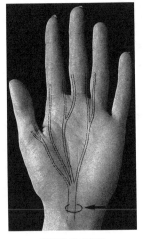

TINEL'S SIGN

Examination Techniques   Possible Findings

o— THE BULGE SIGN
FOR FLUID IN KNEE JOINT.
Milk knee upward to displace
any fluid. Then press behind
lateral edge of patella and
watch for returning fluid.

A bulge of returning fluid indicates fluid within knee
joint. This is a sensitive test
for a small effusion.

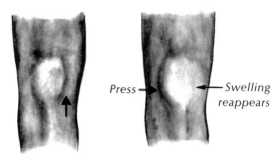

Press — *Swelling
reappears*

Milk upward

o— BALLOON SIGN.
Compress the suprapatellar
pouch with one hand and,
with thumb and finger of the
other, feel for fluid entering
spaces next to patella.

A palpable wave of fluid is a
positive sign, indicating a
fairly large effusion.

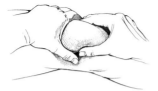

Examination Techniques	**Possible Findings**

o— MEASURING LEG LENGTH. Patient's legs should be aligned symmetrically. With a tape, measure distance from anterior superior iliac spine to medial malleolus. Tape should cross knee medially.

Unequal leg length may be the cause of scoliosis.

ᶜ/o—MEASURING RANGE OF MOTION. To measure range of motion precisely, a simple pocket goniometer is needed. Estimates may be made visually. Movement in the elbow at the right is limited to range indicated by red lines.

A flexion deformity of 45° and further flexion to 90° (45° → 90°).

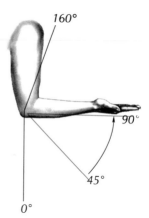

THE NERVOUS SYSTEM

ᶜ   MENTAL STATUS

Recall what you know about the patient's mental status as it relates to the nervous system, and **assess** it further if indicated.

Examination Techniques	Possible Findings

CRANIAL NERVES

CN I (OLFACTORY). Test sense of smell on each side.

Loss in frontal lobe lesions

CN II (OPTIC)

Assess visual acuity.

Blindness

Check visual fields.

Hemianopsia

Inspect optic discs.

Papilledema, optic atrophy

CN II, III (OPTIC AND OCULOMOTOR). **Test** pupillary reactions to light. If they are abnormal, test reactions to near effort.

Blindness, CN III paralysis, tonic pupils, Horner's syndrome may affect light reactions

CN III, IV, VI (OCULOMOTOR, TROCHLEAR, AND ABDUCENS). **Assess** extraocular movements.

Strabismus from paralysis of CN III, IV, or VI; nystagmus

CN V (TRIGEMINAL)

Feel the contractions of temporal and masseter muscles.

Motor or sensory loss from lesions of CN V or its higher motor pathways

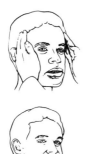

Examination Techniques   **Possible Findings**

Check corneal reflexes.

Test pain and light touch sensations on face.

CN VII (FACIAL). **Ask** patient to raise both eyebrows, frown, close eyes tightly, show teeth, smile, and puff out cheeks.

Weakness from lesion of peripheral nerve, as in Bell's palsy, or of central nervous system, as in a stroke

CN VIII (ACOUSTIC). **Assess** hearing. If it is decreased—

* Test for lateralization (**Weber test**).

* Compare air and bone conduction (**Rinne test**).

Sensorineural loss causes lateralization to less affected ear and AC > BC. Conduction loss causes lateralization to more affected ear and BC > AC.

CN IX, X (GLOSSOPHARYNGEAL AND VAGUS)

Observe any difficulty in swallowing.

A weakened palate or pharynx impairs swallowing.

Listen to the voice.

Hoarse or nasal voice

Watch soft palate rise with "ah."

Palatal paralysis

Test gag reflex on each side.

Absent reflex

Examination Techniques	**Possible Findings**

CN XI (SPINAL ACCESSORY)

- Trapezius muscles. Assess muscles for bulk, involuntary movements, and strength of shoulder shrug.

  Atrophy, fasciculations, weakness

- Sternomastoid muscles. Assess strength as head turns against your hand.

  Weakness

CN XII (HYPOGLOSSAL)

Listen to patient's articulation.

Dysarthria from damage to CN X or CN XII

Inspect the resting tongue.

Atrophy, fasciculations

Inspect the protruded tongue.

Deviation to weak side

℞ THE MOTOR SYSTEM

BODY POSITION

Hemiplegic posture

INVOLUNTARY MOVEMENTS. If movements are present, **observe** their location, quality, rate, rhythm, amplitude, and setting.

Tremors, fasciculations, tics, chorea, athetosis, oral–facial dyskinesias

MUSCLE BULK. **Inspect** muscle contours.

Atrophy

MUSCLE TONE. **Assess** resistance to passive stretch of arms and legs.

Spasticity, rigidity, flaccidity

Examination Techniques

Possible Findings

MUSCLE STRENGTH in major muscle groups:

- Elbow flexion (C5, C6)

- Elbow extension (C6, C7, C8)

- Wrist extension (C6, C7, C8, radial nerve)

- Grip (C7, C8, T1)

- Finger abduction (C8, T1, ulnar nerve)

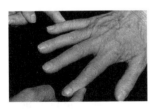

- Thumb opposition (C8, T1, median nerve)

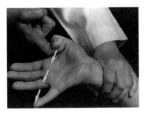

Look for a pattern in any detectable weakness. It may suggest a lower motor lesion affecting a peripheral nerve or nerve root. Weakness of one side of body suggests an upper motor neuron lesion. A polyneuropathy causes symmetrical distal weakness, and a myopathy usually causes proximal weakness. Weakness that worsens with repeated effort and improves with rest suggests myasthenia gravis.

Examination Techniques	Possible Findings

- Trunk—flexion, extension, lateral bending

- Hip flexion (L2, L3, L4)

- Hip adduction (L2, L3, L4)

- Hip abduction (L4, L5, S1)

- Hip extension (S1)

- Knee extension (L2, L3, L4)

- Knee flexion (L4, L5, S1, S2)

- Ankle dorsiflexion (L4, L5)

- Ankle plantar flexion (S1)

Scale for Grading Muscle Strength:

0 No muscular contraction detected

1 A barely detectable trace of contraction

2 Active movement with gravity eliminated

3 Active movement against gravity

Examination Techniques	Possible Findings

4 Active movement
against gravity and some
resistance

5 Active movement
against full resistance

COORDINATION. **Check:**

Rapid alternating movements
in arms and legs

Clumsy, slow movements in
cerebellar disease

Point-to-point movements in
arms and legs

Clumsy, unsteady move-
ments in cerebellar disease

Gait. **Ask** patient to

- Walk away, turn, and
come back

- Walk heel-to-toe

- Walk on toes, then on
heels

- Hop in place on each foot

- Do one-legged shallow
knee bends

Upper or lower motor neu-
ron weakness, cerebellar
ataxia, parkinsonism, and
loss of position sense may all
affect performance.

(Substitute rising from a
chair and climbing on a stool
for hops and bends as indicated.)

Stance

- **Do** a *Romberg Test* (a sensory test of stance). **Ask**
patient to stand with feet
together and eyes open,

Loss of balance that appears
when eyes are closed is a
positive Romberg test, suggesting poor position sense.

Examination Techniques	**Possible Findings**

then closed for 20–30 seconds. Mild swaying may occur. (Stand close by to prevent falls.)

- **Look** for a *pronator drift.* Watch as patient holds arms forward, with eyes closed, for 20–30 seconds.

Flexion and pronation at elbow and downward drift of arm in hemiplegia

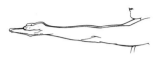 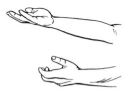

Ask patient to keep arms up, and **tap** them downward. A smooth return to position is normal.

Weakness, incoordination, poor position sense

THE SENSORY SYSTEM

METHODS OF TESTING

Compare symmetrical areas on the two sides of the body.

Hemisensory deficits

Also **compare** distal and proximal areas of arms and legs for *pain, temperature, and touch sensation.* Scatter stimuli to sample most dermatomes and major peripheral nerves.

Glove-and-stocking loss of peripheral neuropathy

Examination Techniques	Possible Findings

Check fingers and toes distally for *vibration and position senses*. If responses are abnormal, test more proximally.

Loss of position and vibration senses in posterior column disease

Map any area of abnormal response.

Except when you are explaining the tests, patient's eyes should be closed.

Assess response to the following stimuli:

- *Pain.* Use the sharp end of a pin or other suitable tool. The dull end serves as a control.

  Analgesia, hypalgesia, hyperalgesia

- *Temperature* (if indicated). Use test tubes with hot and ice-cold water (or other objects of suitable temperature).

  Temperature and pain senses usually correlate with each other.

- *Light touch.* Use a fine wisp of cotton.

  Anesthesia, hyperesthesia

- *Vibration.* Use a 128-Hz or 256-Hz tuning fork, held on a bony prominence.

  Vibration and position senses, both carried in the posterior columns, often correlate with each other.

Examination Techniques   **Possible Findings**

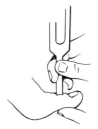

- *Position.* Holding patient's finger or big toe by its sides, move it up or down.

Also **assess** one or more of the *discriminative* sensations:

- *Stereognosis.* Ask for identification of a common object placed in patient's hand.

- *Number identification.* Ask for identification of a number drawn on patient's palm with blunt end of a pen.

Stereognosis, number identification, and two-point discrimination may be impaired by lesions in the posterior columns or in the sensory cortex.

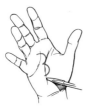

- *Two-point discrimination.* Find minimal distance on pad of patient's finger at which the sides of two points can be distinguished from one (normally <5 mm).

- *Point localization.* Touch skin briefly, and ask patient to open both eyes and identify the place touched.

A lesion in the sensory cortex may impair point localization on the opposite side and cause extinction of the touch sensation on that side.

- *Extinction.* Simultaneously touch opposite, corresponding areas of the body, and ask patient where the touch is felt.

Examination Techniques   **Possible Findings**

REFLEXES

- Biceps (C5, C6)

Hyperactive deep tendon reflexes, absent abdominal reflexes, and a Babinski response indicate an upper motor neuron lesion.

- Triceps (C6, C7)

- Supinator (brachioradialis) (C5, C6)

- Abdominals

Abdominal reflexes may be absent with upper or lower neuron lesions.

Examination Techniques	**Possible Findings**

Upper (T8, T9, T10)

Lower (T10, T11, T12)

 • Knee (L2, L3, L4)

• Ankle (S1)

Ankle jerks symmetrically decreased or absent in peripheral polyneuropathy

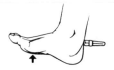

• Plantar (L5, S1), normally flexor

Babinski response

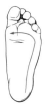   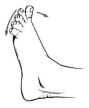

Check for clonus if reflexes seem hyperactive

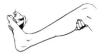

Examination Techniques	**Possible Findings**

Reinforce absent reflexes by isometric contraction of unrelated muscles.

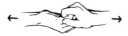

Scale for Grading Reflexes

4+ Hyperactive, with clonus

3+ Brisker than average, not necessarily abnormal

2+ Average, normal

1+ Diminished, low normal

0   No response

SPECIAL TECHNIQUES

WINGING. Ask patient to push against the wall or your hand with a partially straightened arm. Inspect the scapula. It should stay close to the chest wall.

Winging of scapula away from the chest wall suggests weakness of the serratus anterior muscle.

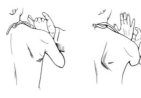

Examination Techniques	**Possible Findings**

ANAL REFLEX. With a dull object, stroke outward from anus in four quadrants. Watch for anal contraction.

Loss of reflex suggests lesion at S 2-3-4 level.

ASTERIXIS. Ask the patient to hold both arms forward, with hands cocked up and fingers spread. Watch for 1–2 minutes.

Sudden brief flexions suggest a metabolic encephalopathy.

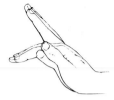

MENINGEAL SIGNS. With patient supine, flex head and neck toward chest. Note resistance or pain, and watch for flexion of hips and knees (**Brudzinski's sign**).

Meningeal irritation may cause resistance to and pain on flexion during both these maneuvers.

Flex one of patient's legs at hip and knee, then straighten knee. Note resistance or pain (**Kernig's sign**).

A compressed lumbosacral nerve root also causes pain on straightening the knee of a raised leg.

ASSESSING THE STUPOROUS OR COMATOSE PATIENT. **Assess** ABCs (airway, breathing, and circulation).

Take pulse, blood pressure, and rectal temperature.

Examination Techniques	Possible Findings
Establish level of consciousness with escalating stimuli.	Lethargy, obtundation, stupor, coma
Don't dilate pupils, and **don't flex** patient's neck if cervical cord may have been injured.	

Observe

• Breathing pattern	Cheyne–Stokes, ataxic breathing
• Pupils	Pinpoint, midposition, one dilated and fixed
• Ocular movements	Deviation to one side
Note posture of body.	Decorticate rigidity, decerebrate rigidity, flaccid hemiplegia

Test for flaccid paralysis.

• Hold the forearms vertically and note wrist positions.	A flaccid hand droops to the horizontal.
• From 12–18 inches above bed, drop each arm.	A flaccid arm drops more rapidly.
• Support both knees in a somewhat flexed position, and then extend each knee and let lower leg drop to the bed.	The flaccid leg drops more rapidly.
• From a similar starting position, release both legs.	A flaccid leg falls into extension and external rotation.

Examination Techniques   **Possible Findings**

Check for the *oculocephalic reflex (doll's-eye movements)*. Holding upper eyelids open, turn head quickly to each side, then flex and extend patient's neck. This patient's head will be turned to her right.

In a comatose patient with an intact brainstem, the eyes move in the opposite direction, in this case to her left (doll's-eye movements).

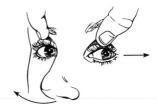

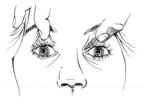

Very deep coma or a lesion in midbrain or pons abolishes this reflex.

Complete the neurologic and general physical examination.

CHAPTER 3

THE EXAMINATION OF INFANTS AND CHILDREN

Bates, B. A POCKET GUIDE TO PHYSICAL EXAMINATION AND HISTORY
TAKING, SECOND EDITION. © 1995 J.B. Lippincott Company.

OVERVIEW

While most of the techniques used to examine adults are applicable to infants and children, there are methods of examination that are unique during infancy (the first year of life), early childhood (1–4 years), and late childhood (5–12 years). Those for which there are differences in methodology will be described here, following the outline for each of the sections of Chapter 2, The Physical Examination of an Adult. Where no differences exist, no comment will be made. The physical examination of adolescents (13–20 years) is conducted essentially as that of the adult.

SEQUENCE OF A COMPREHENSIVE EXAMINATION

Positions for various parts of the examination during infancy and early childhood need not necessarily follow those recommended for examining adults. Some parts can be conducted on the parent's or your lap with the baby supine or sitting. The supine position on the examining table is essential for examination of the abdomen, hips, genitalia, and rectum, and of the mouth and the ears when the baby is resisting.

| **Examination Techniques** | **Possible Findings** |

Infancy and Early Childhood.
No special sequence except
that oral and ear examination, abduction of the hips,
and the rectal examination
(if needed) should be saved
until last, since these usually
cause the baby to cry. Be op-
portunistic and listen to the
heart and lungs and palpate
the abdomen when the baby
is quiet.

Late Childhood. Use the same
order of examination as with
adults, except examine the
most painful areas last.

MENTAL AND PHYSICAL STATUS

Infancy. **Observe** the parents' affect in talking about
their baby, their manner of
holding, moving, and dressing the baby, and their response to situations that
may produce discomfort for
the baby. **Observe** a breast
or bottle feeding.

Normal parental bonding to
the infant. Maladaptive parental nurturing as a cause
of malnutrition and "failure
to thrive"

Determine attainment of
developmental milestones
using the Denver Develop-
mental Screening Test be-
fore conducting the physical
examination.

Normal development versus
delays in personal-social,
fine motor-adaptive, lan-
guage, and gross motor development

Examination Techniques	**Possible Findings**

Early Childhood. **Observe** during the interview the degree of sickness or wellness, mood, state of nutrition, speech, cry, facial expression, apparent chronological and emotional age, developmental skills, and parent–child interaction, including the amount of separation tolerance, displays of affection, and response to discipline.

Normal or abnormal level of general health and development. Parents who abuse their children often pay little attention to them; abused children usually demonstrate no anxiety when separated from their parents.

Late Childhood. **Determine** the child's orientation to time and place, factual knowledge, and language and number skills. **Observe** motor skills used in writing, tying shoelaces, buttoning, using scissors, and drawing.

Normal or abnormal performance, the latter suggesting intellectual impairment or motor disability

THE GENERAL SURVEY

Measurements of vital signs and body size in infants and children often provide the first and only indicators of disease.

Sepsis, chronic renal failure, congenital heart disease, parental deprivation

HEIGHT AND WEIGHT

Growth, reflected in increases in body height and weight within expected limits, is probably the best indicator of health during infancy and childhood. **Plot** each child's height and

Growth measures above the 97th or below the 3rd percentile, or if there has been a recent rise or fall from prior levels, require investigation.

Examination Techniques	**Possible Findings**

weight on standard growth charts to determine if normal progress is being made. See standard grids on pp. 123–126.

HEAD CIRCUMFERENCE

Determine the head circumference at every physical examination during the first 2 years and at least biennially thereafter. See standard grids on pp. 127–128.

Microcephaly, premature closure of the sutures, hydrocephalus, subdural hematoma, brain tumor

With the patient supine, **place** a cloth, soft plastic, or disposable paper centimeter tape over the occipital, parietal, and frontal prominences of the head.

Individual and/or serial measurements of the head circumference are essential for determination of retarded and overly rapid growth of the head.

Stretch the tape and **note** the reading, being sure that the greatest circumference is obtained.

SPECIAL TECHNIQUE

FLUSH TECHNIQUE FOR MEASURING BLOOD PRESSURE (in infants and children <3 years of age). With cuff in place, wrap an elastic bandage snugly around the elevated arm, proceeding from fingers to antecubital space. Inflate cuff to a pressure above the expected systolic reading.

Examination Techniques	Possible Findings
Remove bandage and place the pallid arm at patient's side. Allow pressure to fall slowly until flush of color returns to forearm, hand, and fingers.	When flushing occurs, the sphygmomanometer reading will indicate a blood pressure value somewhere between systolic and diastolic levels.

THE SKIN

Infancy. **Look** for

• Pallor	Anoxia, anemia
• Vasomotor changes	Mottled appearance common in prematurity, cretinism, Down's syndrome
• Cyanosis	Acrocyanosis, congenital heart disease
• Melanotic pigmentation	Mongolian spots
• Jaundice	Sepsis, hemolytic disease, biliary obstruction
• Erythema	Miliaria rubra, erythema toxicum, capillary hemangioma, port-wine stain

THE HEAD

Infancy. **Palpate** the	Head small with microcephaly, enlarged with hydrocephaly
• Anterior and posterior fontanelles	Fontanelles full and tense with meningitis

Examination Techniques	Possible Findings
• Sagittal, coronal, and lambdoidal sutures	Closed with microcephaly. Separated with increased intracranial pressure (hydrocephaly, subdural hematoma, and brain tumor)
• Cranial bones	Swelling due to subperiosteal hemorrhage (cephalhematoma) does not cross suture lines; swelling due to bleeding associated with a fracture does.
Early and Late Childhood. **Auscultate** the skull.	A bruit in a nonanemic child suggests increased intracranial pressure or an intracranial arteriovenous shunt.

S P E C I A L   T E C H N I Q U E S

MACEWEN'S SIGN. Percuss the parietal bone on each side by tapping your index or middle finger directly against its surface.

A "cracked pot" sound is heard prior to closure of the sutures and when increased intracranial pressure causes closed sutures to separate (e.g., in lead encephalopathy and brain tumor).

TRANSILLUMINATION OF THE SKULL. In a completely darkened room, place a standard three-battery flashlight, with a soft rubber collar attached to the lighted end, flush against the skull at various points. Normally, a 2-cm halo of light is present around the circumference of the flash-

Uniform transillumination of the entire head occurs when the cerebral cortex is partially absent or thinned. Localized bright spots may be seen with subdural effusion and porencephalic cysts.

Examination Techniques	**Possible Findings**

light over the frontoparietal area, and a 1-cm halo over the occipital area.

CHVOSTEK'S SIGN. Percuss the top of the cheek just below the zygomatic bone in front of the ear, using the tip of your index or middle finger.

One or two contractions of the facial muscles may occur normally during infancy and early childhood. Repeated contractions occur in tetanus and in tetany due to hypocalcemia and hyperventilation.

THE EYES

Infancy. **Test** for vision by shining a bright light into the eye or moving an object quickly toward it.

Blinking of the eyes and extension of the head will occur if the baby can see.

Early and Late Childhood. **Test** vision of children over age 3 years with the Snellen E chart. Most youngsters will indicate the direction of the E, either orally or by pointing. Normal visual acuity is about 20/40 at age 3 years, 20/30 at age 4 years, and 20/20 at age 6–7 years.

Any difference in visual acuity between the eyes (e.g., 20/20 on left and 20/30 on right) is abnormal, might lead to amblyopia, and should be referred to an ophthalmologist.

S P E C I A L   T E C H N I Q U E

EXAMINATION OF AN INFANT'S EYES. Hold the baby upright, grasping the axillae with your hands and fixing the head with your

The eyes look in the direction you are turning. When the rotation stops, the eyes look in the opposite direction.

| **Examination Techniques** | **Possible Findings** |

thumbs. Extend your arms and rotate yourself with the baby slowly in one direction. The baby's eyes will open, providing a clear view of the scleras, irises, and extraocular movements.

THE EARS

THE AURICLE

Infancy. **Note** whether the upper portion of the newborn's auricle joins the scalp below a line drawn across the inner canthus and outer canthus of the eye.

Auricles that join the scalp below this line suggest the presence of renal agenesis.

THE EAR CANAL AND EARDRUM

Infancy. **Look** at the eardrum with your otoscope by pulling the pinna downward.

The light reflex on the tympanic membrane is diffuse and does not become cone-shaped until several months after birth.

HEARING

Infancy. **Make** a loud, sharp noise near the infant's ear and **watch** for blinking of the eyes (**acoustic blink reflex**).

Absence may indicate decreased hearing.

S P E C I A L   T E C H N I Q U E

PNEUMATIC OTOSCOPY. Place the speculum of a pneumatic otoscope far enough into the external ear

When air is introduced the tympanic membrane moves inward, and when air is removed the membrane

Examination Techniques	Possible Findings

canal to provide a relatively tight air seal. Introduce or remove air from the canal by applying positive and negative pressures with a rubber squeeze bulb attached to the otoscope.

moves outward. This movement is absent in serous otitis media, and diminished in some cases of acute otitis media.

THE NOSE, MOUTH, PHARYNX, AND NECK

NOSE

Infancy. **Test** patency of the nasal passages by occluding each nostril alternately while holding infant's mouth closed.

The baby will be unable to breathe when choanal atresia is present.

MOUTH

Early and Late Childhood. **Ask** child to bite down as hard as possible. **Part** the lips and **observe** alignment of maxilla and mandible.

Normally, the upper teeth slightly override the lower teeth. Overbite and underbite can be detected this way.

PHARYNX

Examine the throat. **Note** size and appearance of tonsils. They are relatively larger in early and late childhood than in infancy and adolescence. They usually have deep crypts on their surfaces, often with white concretions or food particles protruding from their depths—no indication of current or past disease.

A white exudate on the tonsils suggests streptococcal tonsillitis. A thick, gray, adherent exudate suggests diphtheritic tonsillitis. Necrosis (grayish discoloration of the tissue itself) suggests infectious mononucleosis. One red tonsil protruding forward and medially strongly indicates a peritonsillar abscess.

Examination Techniques	**Possible Findings**

NECK

Infancy. **Inspect** and **palpate** the newborn's neck for skin tags, fistulas, masses, cysts, muscle spasm, and crepitus.

Thyroglossal duct fistula or cyst, branchial cleft fistula or cyst, and sternomastoid muscle injury and fractured clavicle from birth trauma

THE THORAX AND LUNGS

Infancy

- **Note** the breathing pattern.

  Alternating rapid (30–40/min) and slow (5–10/min) respirations are considered normal ("periodic") breathing. Apnea (>20 sec) with cardiopulmonary or CNS disease or with high risk for sudden infant death syndrome (SIDS)

- **Note** head movement with breathing.

  Extension of head on inspiration with severe respiratory disease

- **Auscultate** the chest with the bell or small diaphragm, listening for breath sounds.

  Rarely absent, even with atelectasis, effusion, empyema, or pneumothorax. Inspiratory wheeze with narrowing of upper airway, expiratory wheeze with narrowing of lower airway. Fine crackles normally heard at the end of deep inspiration

Examination Techniques	Possible Findings

THE BREASTS

BREASTS

Infancy. **Look** for enlargement of the newborn's breasts with white discharge from nipples.

Normal maternal estrogenic effect lasting several days

Late Childhood. **Look** for asymmetry of breast size in females.

Usual during preadolescence

THE CARDIOVASCULAR SYSTEM

THE ARTERIAL PULSE

Palpate the femoral pulses.

Diminution (as compared to radial pulse) or absence with coarctation of the aorta

BLOOD PRESSURE

For measurement of blood pressure in children under 3 years of age, see the flush method, pp. 98–99. For normal and abnormal levels of blood pressure in children, see pp. 164–165.

THE HEART

Look and **palpate** for the apical pulse.

At 4th interspace until age 7 years, at 5th interspace thereafter. To left of midclavicular line until age 4 years, at MCL ages 4 to 6 years, and to right of MCL after age 7 years.

Examination Techniques	Possible Findings

THE ABDOMEN

Infancy. **Inspect** the newborn's umbilical cord.

There should be two thick-walled arteries and one thin-walled vein. A single umbilical artery suggests the presence of a variety of congenital anomalies.

S P E C I A L   T E C H N I Q U E S

EXAMINATION FOR PYLORIC STENOSIS. Place unclothed infant supine and stand at foot of examining table. Direct a bright light at table height across the abdomen from infant's right side. Feed baby a bottle of sugar water and observe abdomen closely.

With pyloric stenosis, peristaltic waves are seen going across the upper abdomen from left to right with increasing amplitude and frequency until infant vomits with projectile force.

After vomiting occurs, palpate deeply in right upper quadrant with baby supine and then prone, using your extended middle finger.

The hypertrophied pyloric muscle about 2 cm in diameter will be felt.

SCRATCH TEST TO DETERMINE LIVER SIZE. Place diaphragm of stethoscope just above right costal margin at midclavicular line. With your fingernail, lightly scratch skin of abdomen along the midclavicular line, moving from below umbilicus toward costal margin. Listen for the scratching sound.

When the fingernail reaches the liver's lower edge, the sound of scratching will first be heard as it is transmitted through the liver.

Examination Techniques	**Possible Findings**

MALE GENITALIA

HERNIAS

Early and Late Childhood. **Ask** the child to try to lift the chair in which you are sitting.

This will help you to detect inguinal and femoral hernias not discovered when the child was asked to cough or strain down.

S P E C I A L   T E C H N I Q U E

DETECTION OF PSEUDO-UNDESCENDED TESTICLE. Because the cremasteric reflex is so strong during early and late childhood, you may not be able to feel a testicle while examining the scrotum with the child upright or supine. To check for a truly undescended testicle, sit the child cross-legged and palpate the inguinal canal and scrotum.

This positioning interrupts the cremasteric reflex and allows the testicle to descend into the scrotum.

FEMALE GENITALIA

Examine the *female genitalia* while the patient is in the supine frog-leg position. Separate the labia majora at their midpoint with the thumb of each hand applying traction laterally and posteriorly. Inspect the *urethral orifice* and the *vestibule,* defined by the labia minora laterally, the clitoris anteriorly, and the posterior fourchette. Look

Enlargement of clitoris and posterior fusion of labia majora are signs of *ambiguous genitalia*. When present, it is essential to determine the sex of the child before a definite sex assignment is made.

Fusion of labia minora is seen occasionally in girls under 4 years of age. It may be par-

Examination Techniques	Possible Findings
for the *hymen,* a thickened, avascular structure with a central orifice that covers the vaginal opening.	tial, with only the posterior portion of the labia fused, or it may be complete. A thin membrane that joins the labial edges is easily lysed with a cotton swab.

THE MUSCULOSKELETAL SYSTEM

Screening

Observe the child

• Standing upright with feet together	Foot deformities, bow legs, knock-knees, scoliosis
• Walking and running	Limp and other gait abnormalities due to muscle weakness or spasticity
• Stooping to pick up an object	Eye–hand coordination and muscle balance
• Rising from a supine position on the floor	General neurologic integrity and the proximal leg muscle weakness of muscular dystrophy (**Gower's sign**)

THE SPINE

Inspect and **palpate** the lumbosacral spine carefully.

• **Look** and **feel** for defects of the vertebral bodies.	Defects (spina bifida occulta) may be associated with an underlying spinal cord anomaly (diastematomyelia).

Examination Techniques	Possible Findings

- **Look** for abnormalities of the skin, pigmented spots, hairy patches, or deep pits that might overlie external openings of sinus tracts that extend to the spinal canal.

A sinus tract provides potential entry to the spinal canal of organisms that can cause meningitis.

SPECIAL TECHNIQUES

ORTOLANI TEST. With infant supine, legs pointing toward you, flex legs to 90° at hips and knees. Place your index fingers over the greater trochanters of the femurs and your thumbs over the lesser trochanters. Abduct both hips simultaneously until lateral aspect of each knee touches examining table.

When a congenitally dislocated hip is present in a newborn, a click is heard or felt as the femoral head enters the acetabulum near the end of abduction (**Ortolani's sign**). In older infants, decreased abduction of the affected hip(s) may be the only finding of dislocation.

TRENDELENBURG TEST. Observe patient from behind as weight is shifted from one leg to the other.

Note if the pelvis remains level (**negative Trendelenburg sign**) or tilts toward the opposite side (**positive sign**).

A positive Trendelenburg sign is present in diseases of the hip associated with gluteus medius muscle weakness.

Examination Techniques   **Possible Findings**

THE NERVOUS SYSTEM

REFLEXES

Infancy. Because the cortico-spinal pathways are not fully developed at birth, the spinal reflex mechanisms are variable during infancy.

- *Triceps*—Usually not present until after 6 months

- *Abdominals*—Absent at birth, but appear within 6 months

- *Ankle*—Unsustained ankle clonus (8–10 beats) is normal.

  Sustained ankle clonus suggests severe CNS disease.

- *Plantar*—Babinski response present in some (<10%) normal newborns and may remain for as long as 2 years

INFANTILE AUTOMATISMS

Specific reflex activities that test brainstem and spinal cord functions are found in newborns and disappear in early infancy.

Presence or absence of these reflexes does not predict immediate or eventual cortical function positively or negatively. However, absence in the newborn or their persistance beyond their expected time of disappearance suggests severe CNS disease.

PALMAR GRASP REFLEX—disappears at 3 to 4 months

Examination Techniques	Possible Findings
With baby's head in the midline position and arms semiflexed, **place** your index fingers from the ulnar side into baby's hands and **press** against palmar surfaces.	The baby responds by flexing all of its fingers to grasp your fingers.
ROOTING REFLEX—disappears at 3 to 4 months; may be present longer during sleep	
With baby's head in the midline position and hands resting on the anterior chest, **stroke** with your forefinger skin at corners of mouth.	Mouth opens and the head turns to the stroked side.
Stroke middle of upper lip.	Mouth opens and head extends.
Stroke middle of lower lip.	Mouth opens and chin drops.
TRUNK INCURVATION (GALANT'S) REFLEX—disappears at 2 months	
Suspend baby prone in one of your hands.	
Stimulate one side of baby's back approximately 1 cm from the midline along a paravertebral line extending from shoulder to buttocks.	The trunk curves toward the stimulated side with movement of shoulders and pelvis in that direction.
VERTICAL SUSPENSION POSITIONING—disappears after 4 months	

Examination Techniques	**Possible Findings**

Hold baby upright facing away from you with your hands under the axillae.

Normally, head is maintained in the midline and legs flex at hips and knees. Fixed extension and crossed adduction of the legs (scissoring) indicate spastic paraplegia or diplegia.

PLACING RESPONSE—best after 4 days; disappearance time variable

Hold baby upright facing away from you with your hands under the axillae and your thumbs supporting back of head.

Allow dorsal surface of one foot to touch the undersurface of a table top, taking care not to plantar flex the foot. **Repeat** process with other foot.

The foot is lifted reflexly and placed on the table top.

Once both feet are placed on the table top, **propel** the baby forward slowly.

A series of alternate stepping movements of legs and feet occurs.

ROTATION TEST—disappearance time variable

Hold baby upright facing you with your hands under the arms. **Turn** yourself around in one direction and then the other.

Baby's head turns in direction in which you turn.

Restrain baby's head with your thumbs as you turn.

Baby's eyes turn in direction in which you turn.

Examination Techniques	Possible Findings

TONIC NECK REFLEX—may be present at birth, but usually appears at 2 months and disappears at 6 months

With baby supine, **turn** its head to one side and **hold** its chin over its shoulder. Repeat the maneuver, turning the head to the opposite side.

Arm and leg on side to which head is turned extend, while other arm and leg flex. The reflex is considered abnormal when it occurs every time it is evoked.

PEREZ REFLEX—disappears after 3 months

Suspend baby prone in one of your hands. **Press** the thumb of your other hand over the sacrum and **move** it firmly over the spine upward to the neck.

Head and spine extend, knees flex on the abdomen, and baby cries and urinates.

MORO RESPONSE OR STARTLE REFLEX—disappears by 4 months

Hold baby in the supine position, supporting head, back, and legs. Then suddenly **lower** the entire body about 2 feet and **stop** abruptly; or—

Arms abduct briskly and extend at elbows with hands open and fingers extended; legs flex slightly and abduct, but less so than the arms. Arms then come forward over body in a clasping movement, and simultaneously baby cries.

Produce a loud noise (e.g., strike examining table with palms of your hands on both sides of baby's head).

CHAPTER 4

AIDS TO INTERPRETATION

Bates, B. A POCKET GUIDE TO PHYSICAL EXAMINATION AND HISTORY TAKING, SECOND EDITION. © 1995 J.B. Lippincott Company.

LEVELS OF CONSCIOUSNESS

ALERTNESS	Awake, aware of self and environment. When spoken to in a normal voice, patient looks at you and responds fully and appropriately to stimuli.
LETHARGY	When spoken to in a loud voice, patient appears drowsy but opens eyes and looks at you, responds to questions, then falls asleep.
OBTUNDATION	When shaken gently, patient opens eyes and looks at you but responds slowly and is somewhat confused. Alertness and interest in environment decreased.
STUPOR	Patient arouses from sleep only after painful stimuli. Verbal responses slow or absent. Lapses into unresponsiveness when stimulus stops. Minimal awareness of self or environment.
COMA	Despite repeated painful stimuli, patient remains unarousable with eyes closed. No evident response to inner need or external stimuli.

DISORDERS OF SPEECH

APHONIA/ DYSPHONIA

A loss (aphonia) or impairment (dysphonia) of voice due to disease of larynx or its nerve supply. Volume, quality, and pitch of voice affected, as in hoarseness, whisper

DYSARTHRIA

Defective muscular control of lips, tongue, palate, or pharynx, causing nasal, slurred, or indistinct speech. Symbolic aspect of language remains intact. Due to motor lesions in central or peripheral nervous system, parkinsonism, or cerebellar disease

APHASIA

A disorder in producing or understanding language, often due to lesions in the dominant cerebral hemisphere. Two common types:

Wernicke's—Fluent, often rapid, voluble, effortless. Inflection and articulation good, but sentences lack meaning and words are malformed or invented.

Broca's—Nonfluent, slow, effortful, with few words. Inflection and articulation impaired, but words meaningful with nouns, transitive verbs, important adjectives

DELIRIUM AND DEMENTIA

	Delirium	Dementia
TIMING	Acute onset, fluctuating course, lasts hours/weeks	Insidious onset, slowly progressive, lasts months/years
SLEEP PATTERN	Sleep/wake cycle disrupted	Sleep fragmented
MEDICAL ILLNESS OR DRUG TOXICITY	One or both present	Often absent, especially in Alzheimer's disease
LEVEL OF CONSCIOUSNESS	Disturbed. Decreased awareness, attention	Usually normal until late in course
ACTIVITY	Often abnormally decreased or increased	Normal to slow, may be inappropriate
SPEECH	May be slow, hesitant, fast, incoherent	May be aphasic, show difficulty in finding words
MOOD	Labile, may be irritable, fearful, depressed	Often flat, depressed
THOUGHT PROCESSES	Disorganized, may be incoherent	Impoverished, with little information
THOUGHT CONTENT	Delusions common, often transient	Delusions may occur.
PERCEPTIONS	Illusions, hallucinations	Hallucinations may occur.

(continued)

DELIRIUM AND DEMENTIA
(Continued)

	Delirium	Dementia
ORIENTATION	Usually disoriented, especially for time. A known place may seem unfamiliar.	Fairly well maintained, but impaired late in course of illness
ATTENTION	Fluctuates. Person easily distracted, unable to concentrate	Usually not affected until late in illness
CAUSES INCLUDE:	Delirium tremens Uremia Acute liver failure Drug toxicity Hypoxia Hypoglycemia	*Reversible:* Vitamin B_{12} deficiency Thyroid disorders *Irreversible:* Alzheimer's disease Vascular dementia Head trauma

AGE-SPECIFIC HEIGHT/WEIGHT FOR ADULTS (GERONTOLOGY RESEARCH CENTER)

Height*	Weight Range for Men and Women by Age (Years)*				
	20–29	30–39	40–49	50–59	60–69
ft-in		*lb*			
4-10	84–111	92–119	99–127	107–135	115–142
4-11	87–115	95–123	103–131	111–139	119–147
5-0	90–119	98–127	106–135	114–143	123–152
5-1	93–123	101–131	110–140	118–148	127–157
5-2	96–127	105–136	113–144	122–153	131–163
5-3	99–131	108–140	117–149	126–158	135–168
5-4	102–135	112–145	121–154	130–163	140–173
5-5	106–140	115–149	125–159	134–168	144–179
5-6	109–144	119–154	129–164	138–174	148–184
5-7	112–148	122–159	133–169	143–179	153–190
5-8	116–153	126–163	137–174	147–184	158–196
5-9	119–157	130–168	141–179	151–190	162–201
5-10	122–162	134–173	145–184	156–195	167–207
5-11	126–167	137–178	149–190	160–201	172–213
6-0	129–171	141–183	153–195	165–207	177–219
6-1	133–176	145–188	157–200	169–213	182–225
6-2	137–181	149–194	162–206	174–219	187–232
6-3	141–186	153–199	166–212	179–225	192–238
6-4	144–191	157–205	171–218	184–231	197–244

* *Weight without clothes, height without shoes (Andres R, Gerontology Research Center, National Institute on Aging)*

CLASSIFICATION OF A NEWBORN INFANT'S LEVEL OF MATURITY

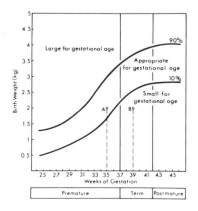

Weight Small for Gestational Age (SGA) = Birth weight < 10th percentile on the intrauterine growth curve

Weight Appropriate for Gestational Age (AGA) = Birth weight within the 10th and 90th percentiles on the intrauterine growth curve

Weight Large for Gestational Age (LGA) = Birth weight > 90th percentile on the intrauterine growth curve

Level of intrauterine growth based on birth weight and gestational age of liveborn, single, white infants. Point A represents a premature infant, while point B indicates an infant of similar birth weight who is mature but small for gestational age; the growth curves are representative of the 10th and 90th percentiles for all of the newborns in the sampling.

(Adapted for publication in the Merck Manual 15th edition, 1987, from Sweet AY: Classification of the low-birth-weight infant. In Klaus MH, Fanaroff AA: Care of the High-Risk Neonate, 3rd ed. Philadelphia, WB Saunders, 1986)

HEIGHT AND WEIGHT GRIDS FOR GIRLS: BIRTH TO 36 MONTHS

GIRLS: BIRTH TO 36 MONTHS
PHYSICAL GROWTH
NCHS PERCENTILES*

NAME _____ RECORD # _____

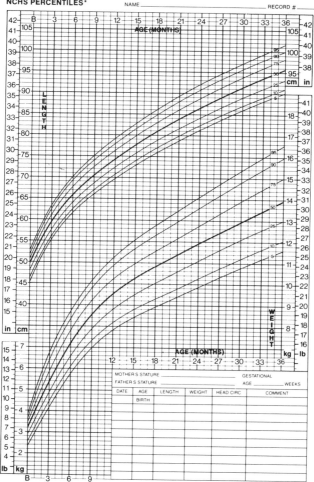

(Adapted from Hamill PVV, Drizd TA, Johnson CL, Reed RB, Roche AF, Moore AM: Physical growth: National Center for Health Statistics percentiles. Am J Clin Nutr 32:607–629, 1979. Data from the National Center for Health Statistics [NCHS], Hyattsville, MD. Figures provided through the courtesy of Ross Laboratories, Columbus, OH)

HEIGHT AND WEIGHT GRIDS FOR GIRLS: 2 TO 18 YEARS

GIRLS: 2 TO 18 YEARS
PHYSICAL GROWTH
NCHS PERCENTILES*

(Adapted from Hamill PVV, Drizd TA, Johnson CL, Reed RB, Roche AF, Moore AM: Physical growth: National Center for Health Statistics percentiles. Am J Clin Nutr 32:607–629, 1979. Data from the National Center for Health Statistics [NCHS], Hyattsville, MD. Figures provided through the courtesy of Ross Laboratories, Columbus, OH)

HEIGHT AND WEIGHT GRIDS FOR BOYS: BIRTH TO 36 MONTHS

BOYS: BIRTH TO 36 MONTHS
PHYSICAL GROWTH
NCHS PERCENTILES*

NAME _____ RECORD # _____

HEIGHT AND WEIGHT GRIDS FOR BOYS: 2 TO 18 YEARS

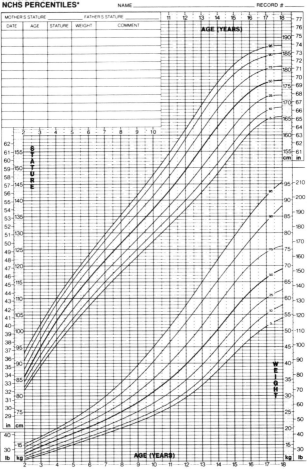

BOYS: BIRTH TO 18 YEARS HEAD CIRCUMFERENCE GROWTH

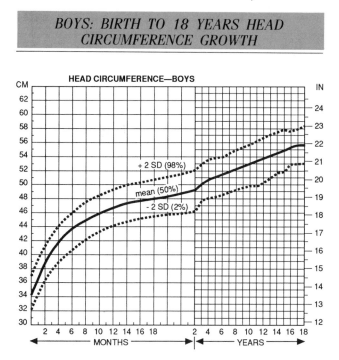

HEAD CIRCUMFERENCE—BOYS

GIRLS: BIRTH TO 18 YEARS HEAD CIRCUMFERENCE GROWTH

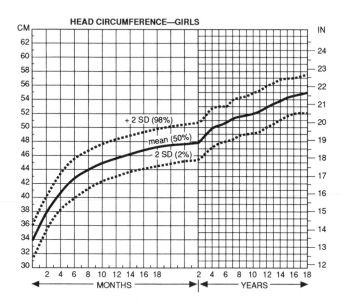

HEAD CIRCUMFERENCE—GIRLS

(Adapted from Nellhaus G: Composite international and interracial graphs. Pediatrics 41:106, 1968)

COLOR CHANGES IN THE SKIN

Color/Mechanism	Selected Causes
BROWN. Increased melanin (greater than a person's genetic norm)	Sun exposure Pregnancy (melasma) Addison's disease
BLUE. (cyanosis) Increased deoxyhemoglobin due to hypoxia:	
• Peripheral	Anxiety or cold environment
• Central (arterial)	Heart or lung disease
Abnormal hemoglobin	Methemoglobinemia, sulfhemoglobinemia
RED. Increased visibility of oxyhemoglobin due to:	
Dilated superifical blood vessels or increased blood flow in skin	Fever, blushing, alcohol intake, local inflammation
Decreased use of oxygen in skin	Cold exposure (e.g., cold ears)
YELLOW	
Increased bilirubin of jaundice (sclera looks yellow)	Liver disease, hemolysis of red blood cells
Carotenemia (sclera does not look yellow)	Increased carotene intake from yellow fruits and vegetables
PALE	
Decreased melanin	Albinism, vitiligo, tinea versicolor
Decreased visibility of oxyhemoglobin due to:	
• Decreased blood flow to skin	Syncope or shock
• Decreased amount of oxyhemoglobin	Anemia
Edema (may mask skin pigments)	Nephrotic syndrome

TYPES OF SKIN LESIONS

Primary Lesions

CIRCUMSCRIBED, FLAT, NONPALPABLE CHANGES IN COLOR

MACULE. Small spot. Examples: freckle, petechia

PATCH. Larger macule. Example: vitiligo

PALPABLE, ELEVATED, SOLID MASSES

PAPULE. Up to 0.5 cm. Example: the papule of acne

PLAQUE. An elevated flat surface larger than 0.5 cm. Example: xanthelasma of the eyelids

NODULE. Larger than 0.5 cm; often deeper and firmer than a papule. Example: epidermoid cyst

TUMOR. Large nodule. Example: a large neurofibroma

WHEAL. A relatively transient, superficial area of local skin edema. Example: mosquito bite

CIRCUMSCRIBED SUPERFICIAL ELEVATIONS OF THE SKIN FORMED BY FREE FLUID IN A CAVITY BETWEEN THE SKIN LAYERS

VESICLE. Up to 0.5 cm; filled with serous fluid. Example: poison ivy

BULLA. Greater than 0.5 cm; filled with serous fluid. Example: 2nd-degree burn

PUSTULE. Filled with pus. Example: acne

(continued)

TYPES OF SKIN LESIONS

Secondary Lesions

LOSS OF SKIN SURFACE

EROSION. Loss of superficial epidermis, leaving a moist area that does not bleed. Example: skin surface after a ruptured vesicle

ULCER. A deeper loss of surface that may bleed and scar. Examples: syphilitic chancre, ulcer of venous insufficiency

FISSURE. A linear crack. Example: athlete's foot

MATERIAL ON THE SKIN SURFACE

CRUST. The dried residue of serum, pus, or blood. Example: a scab

SCALE. A thin flake of exfoliated epidermis. Examples: dry skin, dandruff

FINGERNAILS

CLUBBING

Dorsal phalanx rounded and bulbous; convexity of nail plate increased. Angle between plate and proximal nail fold increased to 180° or more. Proximal nail folds feel spongy. Many causes, including chronic hypoxia and lung cancer

PARONYCHIA

Inflammation of proximal and lateral nail folds, acute or chronic. Folds red, swollen, may be tender

ONYCHOLYSIS

Painless separation of nail plate from nail bed, starting distally. Many causes

TERRY'S NAILS

Whitish with a distal band of reddish brown. Seen in aging and some chronic diseases

LEUKONYCHIA

White spots caused by trauma. They grow out with nail(s).

(continued)

FINGERNAILS

TRANSVERSE WHITE LINES

Curved white lines similar to curve of lunula. They follow an illness and grow out with nails.

BEAU'S LINES

Transverse depressions in nails that follow an illness and grow out with nails

PITTING

Small pits in nail plates. May accompany psoriasis and some other conditions

VISUAL FIELDS

ALTITUDINAL (HORIZONTAL) DEFECT, usually due to a vascular lesion of the retina

UNILATERAL BLINDNESS, due to a lesion of the retina or optic nerve

BITEMPORAL HEMIANOPSIA, due to a lesion of the optic chiasm

HOMONYMOUS HEMIANOPSIA, due to a lesion of the optic tract or optic radiation on the side opposite the blind area

HOMONYMOUS QUADRANTIC DEFECT, due to a partial lesion of the optic radiation on the side opposite the blind area

LEFT   RIGHT

PHYSICAL FINDINGS IN AND AROUND THE EYE

HERNIATED FAT. A common cause of swelling in the lower lid and the inner third of the upper lid; associated with aging

PERIORBITAL EDEMA. Swelling of the eyelids from excessive fluid; many causes

PTOSIS. A drooping upper eyelid that narrows the palpebral fissure; due to a muscle or nerve disorder

ENLARGED PALPEBRAL FISSURE. Due either to retraction of the eyelids or to exophthalmos, both signs of hyperthyroidism

ECTROPION. Outward turning of the margin of the lower lid, exposing the palpebral conjunctiva

 ENTROPION. Inward turning of the lid margin, causing irritation of the cornea or conjunctiva

 PINGUECULAE. Harmless yellowish nodules in the bulbar conjunctiva on either side of the iris; associated with aging

 XANTHELASMA. Yellowish plaques in the eyelids that may be due to a lipid disorder

 BASAL CELL EPITHELIOMA. A common skin cancer

 CHALAZION. A beady nodule in either eyelid due to a chronically inflamed meibomian gland

 STY. A pimplelike infection around a hair follicle near the lid margin

 DACRYOCYSTITIS. An inflammation of the lacrimal sac, acute or chronic, that may obstruct tear drainage

 CORNEAL ARCUS. A grayish white arc or ring often associated with aging

 PTERYGIUM. A thickening of the bulbar conjunctiva that may grow across the cornea

RED EYES

	Pain	Vision	Ocular Discharge	Pupil	Cornea
CONJUNC-TIVITIS	Mild or no discomfort	Only temporary blurring from discharge	Present	Normal	Clear
CILIARY INJECTION					
OF CORNEAL ORIGIN	Present, superficial	Usually decreased	Present	Normal, unless iritis ensues	Varies with cause
ACUTE IRITIS	Present, aching, deep	Decreased	Absent	Small	Clear or slightly clouded
ACUTE GLAUCOMA	Severe, aching, deep	Decreased	Absent	Dilated, fixed	Steamy, cloudy
SUBCONJUNC-TIVAL HEMORRHAGE	Absent	Normal	Absent	Normal	Clear

PUPILLARY ABNORMALITIES

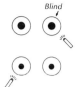
BLIND EYE. Neither a direct nor a consensual response to light occurs when this blind left eye is stimulated. Normal responses occur when the normal right eye is so stimulated.

MARCUS GUNN (DEAFFERENTED) PUPIL. Diminished direct and consensual responses occur when an eye impaired by an optic nerve disorder is stimulated by light. Testing this normal right eye causes normal responses. When the light is swung back to the impaired left eye, the pupils dilate.

HORNER'S SYNDROME. A small pupil due to interruption of its sympathetic nerve supply. Ptosis is associated. Pupillary reactions are normal.

OCULOMOTOR NERVE PARALYSIS. A large pupil, often associated with ptosis of the lid and lateral deviation of the eye. Pupillary reactions absent in that eye

TONIC PUPIL. A large pupil with decreased or absent reaction to light and a slow response to near effort

ARGYLL ROBERTSON PUPILS. Small, irregular pupils that react to near effort but not to light

DILATED FIXED PUPILS. Associated with drug effects or severe brain damage

SMALL FIXED PUPILS. Associated with miotic eye drops, drugs, or brain damage at the level of the pons

RETINAL LESIONS

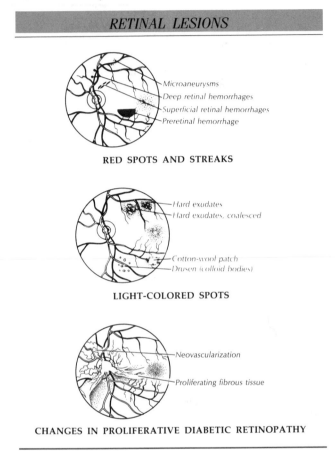

RED SPOTS AND STREAKS

Microaneurysms
Deep retinal hemorrhages
Superficial retinal hemorrhages
Preretinal hemorrhage

LIGHT-COLORED SPOTS

Hard exudates
Hard exudates, coalesced
Cotton-wool patch
Drusen (colloid bodies)

CHANGES IN PROLIFERATIVE DIABETIC RETINOPATHY

Neovascularization
Proliferating fibrous tissue

LUMPS ON OR NEAR THE EAR

CHONDRODERMATITIS HELICIS	Painful, tender, chronic papule on helix or possibly antihelix. May ulcerate and crust
SQUAMOUS CELL CARCINOMA	Growing papule that may ulcerate and crust, most often on helix. Light skin and sun exposure predispose.
EPIDERMOID CYST	A smooth, rounded cyst, often with a dark dot (punctum) that marks the opening of a sebaceous gland. May become inflamed. Often behind the ear
BASAL CELL CARCINOMA	A slow-growing nodule with a lustrous surface and telangiectatic vessels. May ulcerate
LUMPS WITH CHRONIC ARTHRITIS	Consider a rheumatoid nodule that accompanies rheumatoid arthritis or a tophus of chronic tophaceous gout. The latter discharges white chalky crystals of uric acid.
KELOID	A nodular hypertrophic mass of scar tissue that follows injury such as piercing the ears. Darker-skinned people more susceptible
ENLARGED LYMPH NODES	The preauricular and postauricular nodes, when enlarged, may cause lumps beneath the skin in front of and behind the ear respectively.

ABNORMAL EARDRUMS

SEROUS EFFUSION

Fluid level
Air bubble
Amber

Amber fluid behind the eardrum, with or without air bubbles

Associated with viral upper respiratory infections or sudden changes in atmospheric pressure (diving, flying)

ACUTE OTITIS MEDIA

Red, bulging drum, loss of landmarks

Associated with bacterial infection

TYMPANO-SCLEROSIS

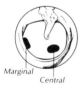

A chalky white patch

Scar of an old otitis media; of little or no clinical consequence

PERFORATION

Marginal   Central

Hole in the eardrum that may be central or marginal

Usually the result of otitis media or trauma

PATTERNS OF HEARING LOSS

	Conductive Loss	Sensorineural Loss
IMPAIRED UNDERSTANDING OF WORDS	Minor	Often troublesome
EFFECT OF NOISY ENVIRONMENT	May help	Increases the hearing difficulty
USUAL AGE OF ONSET	Childhood, young adulthood	Middle and old age
EAR CANAL AND DRUM	Often a visible abnormality	The problem not visible
WEBER TEST (IN UNILATERAL HEARING LOSS)	Lateralizes to the impaired ear	Lateralizes to the good ear
RINNE TEST	BC > AC or BC = AC	AC > BC
CAUSES INCLUDE:	Plugged ear canal, otitis media, immobile or perforated drum, otosclerosis	Sustained loud noise, drugs, inner ear infections, trauma, hereditary disorders, aging

ABNORMALITIES OF THE LIPS

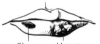

Chance   Herpes

HERPES SIMPLEX. Painful vesicles followed by crusting

SYPHILITIC CHANCRE. A firm lesion that ulcerates and may crust

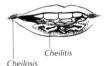

Cheilitis
Cheilosis

ANGULAR STOMATITIS (CHEILOSIS). Softening and cracking at the angles of the mouth

CHEILITIS. Painful cracking, scaling, and crusting of the lower lip

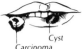

Cyst
Carcinoma

MUCOUS RETENTION CYST. A rounded, soft, often bluish nodule. Benign

CARCINOMA OF THE LIP. A thickened plaque or irregular nodule that may ulcerate or crust. Malignant

PEUTZ–JEGHERS SYNDROME. Brown spots, significant because of their association with intestinal polyposis

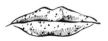

HEREDITARY HEMORRHAGIC TELANGIECTASIA. Red spots, significant because of associated bleeding from nose and GI tract

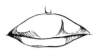

ANGIOEDEMA. Diffuse, tense, subcutaneous swelling, usually allergic in cause

ABNORMALITIES OF THE GUMS AND TEETH

MARGINAL GINGIVITIS. Red, swollen gum margins with blunted interdental papillae

PERIODONTITIS. A progression of gingivitis to deeper tissues, with resulting recession of the gums and looseness or loss of teeth

ACUTE NECROTIZING ULCERATIVE GINGIVITIS. Red, painful gums with marginal ulceration and a grayish pseudomembrane. Foul breath, fever, lymphadenopathy

GINGIVAL ENLARGEMENT. Enlarged gums that partially cover the teeth with heaped-up tissue.

PREGNANCY TUMOR (Pyogenic Granuloma). Red, soft, local mass of enlarged gingiva

DENTAL CARIES. Tooth decay. Clinically invisible in its early stages, it may produce chalky white spots that later discolor to brown or black, soften, and cavitate.

HUTCHINSON'S TEETH. A sign of congenital syphilis, most often involving the upper central incisors. These teeth are small, notched, tapered, and widely spaced.

ABRASION OF TEETH. Irregularities in the biting edges due to recurrent trauma

ATTRITION OF TEETH. Wear of the teeth. The exposed dentin is often yellow or brown.

TONGUES

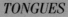

 SMOOTH TONGUE. Due to loss of papillae caused by vitamin B or iron deficiency or possibly anticancer drugs

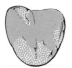 **HAIRY TONGUE.** Due to elongated papillae that may look yellowish, brown, or black. Harmless

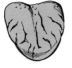 **GEOGRAPHIC TONGUE.** Scattered areas in which the papillae are lost, giving a map-like appearance. Harmless

 FISSURED TONGUE. Fissures may appear with aging. Harmless

 CANDIDA INFECTION. May show a thick, white coat, which when scraped off leaves a raw red surface. Tongue may also be red. Antibiotics, corticosteroids, AIDS may predispose.

 HAIRY LEUKOPLAKIA. White, raised, feathery areas usually on sides of tongue, due to HIV infection, AIDS

HYPOGLOSSAL NERVE PARALYSIS. Atrophy and fasciculations on the involved side, with deviation of the tongue toward it

(continued)

TONGUES

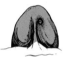

APHTHOUS ULCER (CANKER SORE). Painful, small, whitish ulcer with a red halo. Heals in 7–10 days.

MUCOUS PATCH. Slightly raised, oval lesion, covered by a grayish membrane. Due to secondary syphilis

VARICOSE VEINS (CAVIAR LESIONS). Dark round spots on the undersurface of the tongue, associated with aging

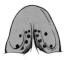

CARCINOMA OF THE TONGUE. A malignancy that should be considered in any nodule or nonhealing ulcer at the base or edges of the tongue

ABNORMALITIES OF THE PHARYNX

Swollen, red

Exudate

EXUDATIVE PHARYNGITIS. A sore red throat with patches of whitish exudate on the tonsils. Is associated with streptococcal pharyngitis and some viral illnesses, including infectious mononucleosis. In diphtheria, unlike streptococcal infections, the exudate may spread as a gray membrane over the soft palate and uvula.

PERITONSILLAR ABSCESS. A unilateral red bulge in the pharynx that may displace the uvula toward the opposite side

UNILATERAL PARALYSIS OF THE VAGUS NERVE. With "ah," the soft palate fails to rise on the involved side and the uvula deviates to the opposite side.

ABNORMALITIES OF THE HARD PALATE

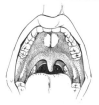

TORUS PALATINUS. A midline bony outgrowth in the hard palate. Size and lobulation vary from person to person.

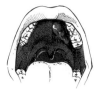

KAPOSI'S SARCOMA. A mass in the palate, especially when not midline, may be a tumor such as Kaposi's sarcoma in AIDS. The classic purple-red color may not be present.

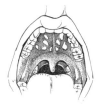

CANDIDA **INFECTION.** White patches that can be scraped off suggest this diagnosis.

ABNORMALITIES OF THE THYROID GLAND

 DIFFUSE ENLARGEMENT. May be due to Graves' disease, Hashimoto's thyroiditis, endemic goiter (iodine deficiency), or sporadic goiter

 MULTINODULAR GOITER. An enlargement with two or more identifiable nodules, usually metabolic in cause

 SINGLE NODULE. May be due to a cyst, a benign tumor, or cancer of the thyroid, or may be one palpable nodule in a clinically unrecognized multinodular goiter

ABNORMALITIES OF THYROID FUNCTION

Hyperthyroidism	Hypothyroidism
Nervousness	Fatigue
Weight loss	Weight gain
Sweating, heat intolerance; skin warm, smooth, moist	Dry skin, cold intolerance, hair loss, nonpitting edema
Frequent stools	Constipation
Tremor, proximal weakness	Weakness; poor memory, hearing
Tachycardia, atrial fibrillation	Bradycardia; hypothermia (late)
In Graves' disease, stare, lid lag, exophthalmos	Periorbital edema

RATE AND RHYTHM OF BREATHING

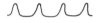

Inspiration Expiration

Time

Volume of air

NORMAL. In adults, 14 to 20 per minute; in infants, up to 44 per minute

〜〜〜〜〜〜〜〜〜〜〜

RAPID SHALLOW BREATHING (TACHYPNEA). Many causes, including restrictive lung disease and pleural pain

〜〜〜〜〜〜

RAPID DEEP BREATHING (HYPERPNEA, HYPERVENTILATION). Many causes, including exercise, anxiety, metabolic acidosis, brainstem injury. *Kussmaul breathing*, due to metabolic acidosis, is deep but rate may be fast, slow, or normal.

〜〜〜〜

SLOW BREATHING. May be due to diabetic coma, drug-induced respiratory depression, increased intracranial pressure

〜〜〜〜

Hyperpnea   Apnea

CHEYNE–STOKES BREATHING. Rhythmically alternating periods of hyperpnea and apnea. In infants and the aged, may be normal during sleep; also accompanies brain damage, heart failure, uremia, and respiratory depression

〜〜〜〜

ATAXIC (BIOT'S) BREATHING. Unpredictable irregularity of depth and rate. Causes include brain damage and respiratory depression.

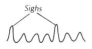

Sighs

SIGHING RESPIRATION. Breathing punctuated by frequent sighs. When associated with other symptoms, it suggests the hyperventilation syndrome. Occasional sighs are normal.

DEFORMITIES OF THE THORAX

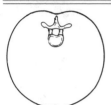

BARREL CHEST. An anteroposterior diameter increased from the adult norm so that the chest (in cross-section) becomes rounded. May accompany aging and chronic obstructive pulmonary disease. (The chest of a normal infant also has this shape.)

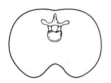

FUNNEL CHEST (PECTUS EXCAVATUM). Posterior displacement of the lower sternum. Compression of the heart or great vessels may cause murmurs.

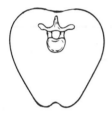

PIGEON CHEST (PECTUS CARINATUM). Anterior displacement of the sternum. The costal cartilages adjacent to the sternum are relatively depressed.

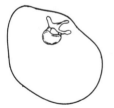

THORACIC KYPHOSCOLIOSIS. A structural spinal curvature that may be associated with distortion and asymmetry of the chest

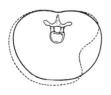

FLAIL CHEST. Abnormal respiratory movements associated with multiple rib fractures. The injured area moves inward in inspiration, outward in expiration.

LUNG LOBES

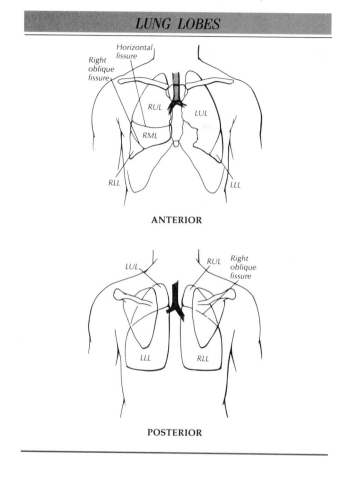

ANTERIOR

POSTERIOR

PERCUSSION NOTES

	Relative Intensity, Pitch, and Duration	Examples
FLATNESS	Soft/high/short	Large pleural effusion
DULLNESS	Medium/medium/medium	Lobar pneumonia
RESONANCE	Loud/low/long	Normal lung, simple chronic bronchitis
HYPERRESONANCE	Louder, lower, longer	Emphysema, pneumothorax
TYMPANY	Loud/high*/*	Large pneumothorax

* Distinguished mainly by musical timbre

BREATH SOUNDS

	Duration	Intensity and Pitch of Expiratory Sound	Example Locations
VESICULAR	Insp > exp	Soft/low	Most of the lungs
BRONCHO-VESICULAR	Insp = exp	Medium/medium	1st and 2nd interspaces, interscapular area
BRONCHIAL	Exp > insp	Loud/high	Over the manubrium; lobar pneumonia
TRACHEAL	Insp = exp	Very loud/high	Over the trachea

In the figures above, duration is indicated by the length of the line, intensity by the width of the line, and pitch by the slope of the line.

TRANSMITTED VOICE SOUNDS

Through Normally Air-Filled Lung	Through Airless Lung*
Spoken words muffled and indistinct	Spoken words louder, clearer (*bronchophony*)
Spoken "ee" heard as "ee"	Spoken "ee" heard as "ay" (*egophony*)
Whispered words faint and indistinct, if heard at all	Whispered words louder, clearer (*whispered pectoriloquy*)
Usually accompanied by vesicular breath sounds and normal tactile fremitus	Usually accompanied by bronchial or bronchovesicular breath sounds and increased tactile fremitus

* As in lobar pneumonia and toward the top of a large pleural effusion

ADVENTITIOUS LUNG SOUNDS

DISCONTINUOUS SOUNDS (CRACKLES). Intermittent, nonmusical, short sounds, like dots in time

- *Fine crackles* (· · · ·) —soft, high in pitch, very brief
- *Coarse crackles* (•••) —somewhat louder, lower in pitch, not quite so brief

CRACKLES CLASSIFIED BY TIMING

- *Late inspiratory crackles.* Must continue into late inspiration. Usually fine, profuse, and heard in dependent portions of the lungs. Causes include interstitial lung disease and early congestive heart failure.

- *Early inspiratory crackles.* Do not continue into late inspiration. Often coarse. Causes include chronic bronchitis and asthma.

CONTINUOUS SOUNDS. Musical and notably longer than crackles, like dashes in time, but not necessarily truly continuous. May be generalized (as in asthma or chronic obstructive lung disease) or persistent and local (as from a tumor or foreign body that is obstructing a bronchus). Clearing by cough or deep breathing suggests secretions as the cause.

- *Wheezes* (〰〰〰)—relatively high in pitch (around 400 Hz or more), with a hissing or shrill quality
- *Rhonchi* (〰〰〰)—relatively low in pitch (around 200 Hz or less), with a snoring quality

STRIDOR. A wheeze heard only or chiefly in inspiration and often louder in the neck than over the chest. Indicates partial airway obstruction in the neck

PLEURAL RUB. A creaking, grating sound associated with respiratory movements. Originates in inflamed pleural surfaces

MEDIASTINAL CRUNCH. A series of precordial crackles synchronous with the heart beat, heard best in the left lateral position. Due to mediastinal emphysema (pneumomediastinum)

SIGNS IN SELECTED

	Trachea	Percussion Note
CHRONIC BRONCHITIS	Midline	Resonant
LEFT HEART FAILURE (EARLY)	Midline	Resonant
CONSOLIDATION*	Midline	Dull
ATELECTASIS (LOBAR)	May be shifted toward	Dull
PLEURAL EFFUSION (LARGE)	May be shifted away	Dull
PNEUMOTHORAX	May be shifted away	Hyperresonant or tympanitic
EMPHYSEMA	Midline	Hyperresonant
ASTHMA	Midline	Normal to hyperresonant

* As in lobar pneumonia, pulmonary edema, or pulmonary hemorrhage

CHEST DISORDERS

Breath Sounds	Transmitted Voice Sounds	Adventitious Sounds
Normal	Normal	None, or wheezes, rhonchi, crackles
Normal	Normal	Late inspiratory crackles in lower lungs; possible wheezes
Bronchial	Increased*	Late inspiratory crackles
Usually absent	Usually absent	None
Decreased to absent	Decreased to absent	Usually none; possible pleural rub
Decreased to absent	Decreased to absent	Possible pleural rub
Decreased to absent	Decreased	None unless bronchitis also
May be obscured by wheezes	Decreased	Wheezes, perhaps crackles

* With increased tactile fremitus, bronchophony, egophony, whispered pectoriloquy

COMMON BREAST NODULES

	Gross Cyst	Fibroadenoma	Cancer
USUAL AGE	30–60 years	Puberty and young adulthood, up to age 55	30–90 years
NUMBER	Single or multiple	Usually single, may be mutliple	Usually single; other nodules may coexist
SHAPE	Round	Round, disclike, or lobular	Irregular or stellate
CONSISTENCY	Soft to firm, usually elastic	May be soft, usually firm	Firm or hard
DELIMITATION	Well circumscribed	Well circumscribed	Not clearly delineated from surrounding tissues
MOBILITY	Mobile	Very mobile	May be fixed
TENDERNESS	Often tender	Usually nontender	Usually nontender
RETRACTION SIGNS	Absent	Absent	May be present

SEX MATURITY RATINGS IN GIRLS: BREASTS

Stage 1

Preadolescent—elevation of nipple only

Stage 2

Stage 3

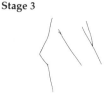

Breast bud stage. Elevation of breast and nipple as a small mound; enlargement of areolar diameter

Further enlargement and elevation of breast and areola, with no separation of the contours

Stage 4

Stage 5

Projection of areola and nipple to form a secondary mound above the level of the breast

Mature stage; projection of nipple only. Areola has receded to general contour of the breast (although in some normal individuals areola continues to form a secondary mound).

(Illustrations through the courtesy of W.A. Daniel, Jr.)

SEX MATURITY RATINGS IN GIRLS: PUBIC HAIR

Stage 1   Preadolescent—no pubic hair except for the fine body hair (vellus hair) similar to that on the abdomen

Stage 2

Stage 3

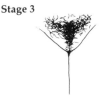

Sparse growth of long, slightly pigmented, downy hair, straight or only slightly curled, chiefly along the labia

Darker, coarser, curlier hair, spreading sparsely over the pubic symphysis

Stage 4

Stage 5

Coarse and curly hair as in adults; area covered greater than in stage 3 but not as great as in the adult and not yet including the thighs

Hair adult in quantity and quality, spread on the medial surfaces of the thighs but not up over the abdomen

(Illustrations through the courtesy of W.A. Daniel, Jr.)

HEART RATES AND RHYTHMS

REGULAR RHYTHMS

FAST (OVER 100)

Sinus tachycardia

Atrial or nodal (supraventricular) tachycardia

Atrial flutter with a regular ventricular response

Ventricular tachycardia

NORMAL (60–100)

Normal sinus rhythm

Second-degree AV block

Atrial flutter with a regular ventricular response

SLOW

Sinus bradycardia

Second-degree AV block

Complete heart block

IRREGULAR RHYTHMS

RHYTHMICALLY OR SPORADICALLY IRREGULAR

Premature contractions (atrial, nodal, or ventricular)

Sinus arrhythmia

TOTALLY IRREGULAR

Atrial fibrillation

Atrial flutter with varying block

AVERAGE HEART RATE OF INFANTS AND CHILDREN AT REST

Age	Average Rate	Range (Two Standard Deviations)
Birth	140	90–190
1st 6 months	130	80–180
6–12 months	115	75–155
1–2 years	110	70–150
2–6 years	103	68–138
6–10 years	95	65–125
10–14 years	85	55–115

BLOOD PRESSURE IN ADULTS

RECOMMENDED SIZE OF THE INFLATABLE BAG

- Width 40% of the arm circumference
- Length 80% of the arm circumference

DIASTOLIC PRESSURE: The disappearance point of Korotkoff sounds in adults, the muffle point in children

METHODS OF INTENSIFYING KOROTKOFF SOUNDS

1. Raise patient's arm before and during inflation; then lower arm and take blood pressure.
2. Inflate cuff, ask patient to make a fist several times, and take blood pressure.

CLASSIFICATION OF BLOOD PRESSURE LEVELS IN ADULTS

Categorize by two or more measurements (averaged) taken on two or more visits after an initial screening.

Category*	Systolic (mm Hg)	Diastolic (mm Hg)
Hypertension		
Very severe	≥210	≥120
Severe	180–209	110–119
Moderate	160–179	100–109
Mild	140–159	90–99
High normal	130–139	85–89
Normal	<130	<85

* *When the systolic and diastolic levels indicate different categories, use the higher category. For example, 170/92 mm Hg is moderate hypertension and 200/120 mm Hg is very severe hypertension.*

In isolated systolic hypertension, *systolic pressure is 140 mm Hg or more and diastolic pressure is less than 90 mm Hg.*

Orthostatic (postural) hypotension: *A decrease of 20 mm Hg or more in systolic pressure, especially when accompanied by symptoms, after the patient changes from the supine to a sitting or standing position*

BLOOD PRESSURE IN CHILDREN

RECOMMENDED SIZE OF THE INFLATABLE BAG

- Width 75% of the upper arm or thigh
- Length 100% or more of the upper arm or thigh circumference

METHOD

Same as for adults in children age 3 years and older

Use flush method for infants and younger children (see pp. 98–99).

CLASSIFICATION OF BLOOD PRESSURE LEVELS IN CHILDREN

NORMAL: Systolic and diastolic BPs < 90th percentile for age and sex

HIGH NORMAL: Average systolic and diastolic BPs between the 90th and 95th percentiles for age and sex

HIGH (HYPERTENSION): Average systolic and/or diastolic BPs ≥ 95th percentile for age and sex

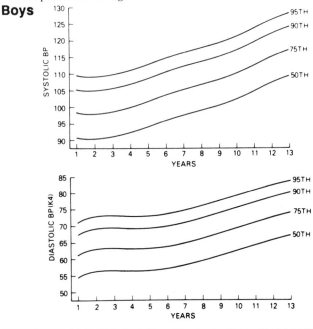

Boys

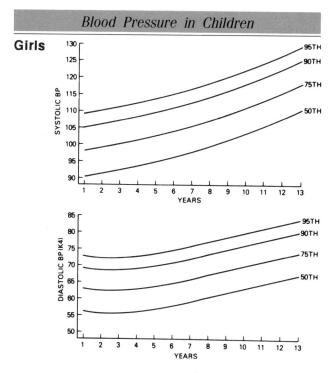

Blood Pressure in Children

Percentiles of BP measurements in boys and girls 1 to 13 years of age.
K4 = Korotkoff phase IV sound (low-pitched and muffled)

(Reproduced with permission from the Second Task Force on Blood
Pressure Control in Children of the National Heart, Lung, and Blood
Institute. Pediatrics [Suppl] 79:1–25, 1987)

THE APICAL IMPULSE

	Normal	Hyperkinetic	Pressure Overload	Volume Overload
LOCATION	5th or 4th left interspace, inside midclavicular line	Normal	Normal	Displaced to the left and possibly downward
DIAMETER	Little more than 2 cm (1 cm in children); ≤3 cm when patient lies on left side	Normal	Increased	Increased
AMPLITUDE	Small, gently tapping	Increased	Increased	Increased
DURATION	Less than ⅔ of systole, stops before S_2	Normal	Prolonged, perhaps up to S_2	Often slightly prolonged
EXAMPLES OF CAUSES		Anxiety, hyperthyroidism, severe anemia	Hypertension, aortic stenosis	Aortic or mitral regurgitation

HEART SOUNDS

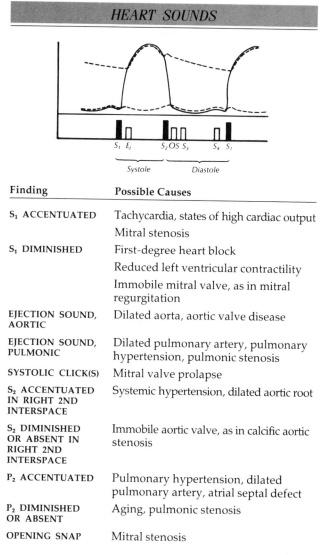

Finding	Possible Causes
S₁ ACCENTUATED	Tachycardia, states of high cardiac output
	Mitral stenosis
S₁ DIMINISHED	First-degree heart block
	Reduced left ventricular contractility
	Immobile mitral valve, as in mitral regurgitation
EJECTION SOUND, AORTIC	Dilated aorta, aortic valve disease
EJECTION SOUND, PULMONIC	Dilated pulmonary artery, pulmonary hypertension, pulmonic stenosis
SYSTOLIC CLICK(S)	Mitral valve prolapse
S₂ ACCENTUATED IN RIGHT 2ND INTERSPACE	Systemic hypertension, dilated aortic root
S₂ DIMINISHED OR ABSENT IN RIGHT 2ND INTERSPACE	Immobile aortic valve, as in calcific aortic stenosis
P₂ ACCENTUATED	Pulmonary hypertension, dilated pulmonary artery, atrial septal defect
P₂ DIMINISHED OR ABSENT	Aging, pulmonic stenosis
OPENING SNAP	Mitral stenosis

(continued)

HEART SOUNDS
(Continued)

Finding	Possible Causes
S_3	Physiologic (usually in children and young adults)
	Pathologic: myocardial failure, volume overload of a ventricle, as in mitral regurgitation
S_4	Excellent physical conditioning (trained athletes)
	Resistance to ventricular filling because of decreased compliance, as in hypertensive artery disease or coronary artery disease

AN APPARENTLY SPLIT FIRST HEART SOUND

	Split S_1	Aortic Ejection Sound	Early Systolic Click	Left-Sided S_4
	‖ I	I I	‖ I	‖ I
BEST HEARD AT	Lower left sternal border	Right 2nd interspace, apex, or both	At or medial to apex or at left sternal border	Apex
PITCH	High	High	High	Low
QUALITY	Both components similar	Clicking	Clicking	Dull
LOUDER WITH	Diaphragm	Diaphragm	Diaphragm	Bell
PALPABLE SPLIT	Absent	Absent	Absent	May be present
AIDS	None	None	Click delayed by squatting	Partial left lateral decubitus position

SPLITTING OF THE SECOND HEART SOUND

PHYSIOLOGIC   Splitting increased in inspiration, usually disappears in expiration, especially if patient sits. A_2 precedes P_2.

WIDE   Splitting persistent through cardiac cycle and increases on inspiration. May be due to delayed P_2 (as in right bundle branch block, pulmonic stenosis) or early A_2 (as in mitral regurgitation)

FIXED   Wide splitting that does not vary with respiration. Occurs in atrial septal defect, right ventricular failure

PARADOXICAL   Splitting that appears on expiration and disappears on inspiration. A_2 is abnormally delayed and follows P_2. Occurs in left bundle branch block

HEART MURMURS AND SIMILAR SOUNDS

Likely Causes

MIDSYSTOLIC

Innocent murmurs (no cardiovascular abnormality)

Physiologic murmurs (from increased flow across a semilunar valve, as in pregnancy, fever, anemia)

Aortic stenosis

Murmurs that mimic aortic stenosis (aortic sclerosis, bicuspid aortic valve, dilated aorta, and pathologically increased systolic flow across the aortic valve)

Hypertrophic cardiomyopathy

Pulmonic stenosis

PANSYSTOLIC

Mitral regurgitation

Tricuspid regurgitation

Ventricular septal defect

LATE SYSTOLIC

Mitral valve prolapse

EARLY DIASTOLIC

Aortic regurgitation

MIDDIASTOLIC AND PRESYSTOLIC

Mitral stenosis

CONTINUOUS MURMURS AND MURMURLIKE SOUNDS

Patent ductus arteriosus

Pericardial friction rub (a scratchy sound with 1–3 components)

Venous hum

CYANOSIS AND CONGENITAL HEART DISEASE

No Cyanosis	Early Cyanosis	Late Cyanosis
Small septal defects		Large septal defects
Mild pure pulmonic stenosis	Severe pulmonic stenosis with intact ventricular system	Mild pure pulmonic stenosis
Coarctation of the aorta	Severe tetralogy of Fallot	Less severe tetralogy of Fallot
Patent ductus arteriosus	Tricuspid atresia	Eisenmenger's complex
Anomalous origin of left coronary artery	Two- and three-chambered hearts	
Subendocardial fibroelastosis	Transposition of the great vessels	
Glycogen storage disease		

TENDER ABDOMENS

Visceral Tenderness   **Peritoneal Tenderness**

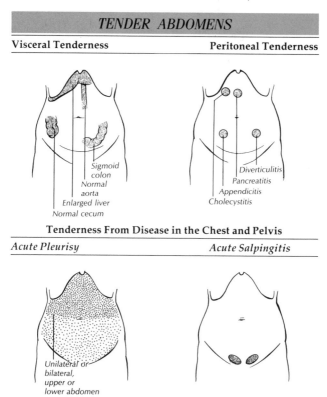

Sigmoid
colon
Normal
aorta
Enlarged liver
Normal cecum

Diverticulitis
Pancreatitis
Appendicitis
Cholecystitis

Tenderness From Disease in the Chest and Pelvis

Acute Pleurisy   *Acute Salpingitis*

Unilateral or
bilateral,
upper or
lower abdomen

SEX MATURITY

In assigning SMRs in boys, observe each of the three characteristics separately. Record two separate ratings: pubic hair and genital. If the penis and testes differ in their stages, average the two into a single figure for the genital rating.

Pubic Hair

Stage 1		Preadolescent—no pubic hair except for the fine body hair (vellus hair) similar to that on the abdomen
Stage 2		Sparse growth of long, slightly pigmented, downy hair, straight or only slightly curled, chiefly at the base of the penis
Stage 3		Darker, coarser, curlier hair spreading sparsely over the pubic symphysis
Stage 4		Coarse and curly hair, as in the adult; area covered greater than in stage 3 but not as great as in the adult and not yet including the thighs
Stage 5		Hair adult in quantity and quality, spread to the medial surfaces of the thighs but not up over the abdomen

(Illustrations through the courtesy of W.A. Daniel, Jr.)

RATINGS IN BOYS

Genital	
Penis	*Testes and Scrotum*
Preadolescent—same size and proportions as in childhood	Preadolescent—same size and proportions as in childhood
Slight to no enlargement	Testes larger; scrotum larger, somewhat reddened, and altered in texture
Larger, especially in length	Further enlarged
Further enlarged in length and breadth, with development of the glans	Further enlarged; scrotal skin darkened
Adult in size and shape	Adult in size and shape

ABNORMALITIES OF THE PENIS

HYPOSPADIAS. Congenital displacement of the urethral meatus to the inferior surface of the penis

PHIMOSIS. A tight prepuce that cannot be retracted

PARAPHIMOSIS. A tight prepuce that, once retracted, cannot be replaced over the glans

BALANITIS. Inflammation of the glans

BALANOPOSTHITIS. Inflammation of the glans and prepuce

CHANCRE. A usually nontender, firm erosion or ulcer, typically on the glans; due to primary syphilis

GENITAL HERPES. A cluster of small vesicles, typically on the glans, that evolve into painful small ulcers on red bases

VENEREAL WARTS. Warty growths on the glans, shaft, or base of the penis; due to human papillomavirus

CANCER OF THE PENIS. An indurated and usually nontender nodule or ulcer of the glans or inner surface of the prepuce. Seen mainly in uncircumcised men

ABNORMALITIES IN THE SCROTUM

SCROTAL HERNIA. Protrusion of abdominal contents through the external inguinal ring into the scrotum. The clinician's fingers cannot get above the mass.

HYDROCELE. A fluid-filled sac in the tunica vaginalis. The clinician's fingers can get above the scrotal mass.

ACUTE ORCHITIS. An acutely tender, swollen testis due to infection

ACUTE EPIDIDYMITIS. A tender, swollen epididymis, usually associated with infection of the urinary tract or prostate

TUBERCULOUS EPIDIDYMITIS. Chronic inflammatory enlargement of the epididymis, often with thickening of the vas deferens

VARICOCELE. Varicose veins of the spermatic cord, traditionally described as feeling like a "bag of worms"

(continued)

ABNORMALITIES IN THE SCROTUM
(Continued)

TUMOR OF THE TESTIS. A usually painless, solid nodule or mass in the testis

CYST OF THE EPIDIDYMIS. A small, painless, fluid-filled mass above the testis. A *spermatocele* is clinically like a cyst but contains sperm.

TORSION OF THE SPERMATIC CORD. An acutely tender, swollen testis due to twisting of the organ on the spermatic cord, with resulting circulatory impairment

SMALL TESTIS. Small, firm testes suggest Klinefelter's syndrome; small, soft testis(es) suggest atrophy.

CRYPTORCHIDISM. An undescended testicle, not palpable in the scrotum. The scrotal sac is poorly developed on the involved side(s). Associated with increased risk of testicular carcinoma.

HERNIAS IN THE GROIN

INDIRECT INGUINAL

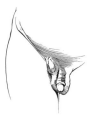

Most common hernia at all ages, both sexes. Originates above inguinal ligament and often passes into scrotum. May touch examiner's fingertip in inguinal canal

DIRECT INGUINAL

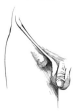

Less common than indirect hernia, usually occurs in men over age 40. Originates above inguinal ligament near external inguinal ring and rarely enters scrotum. May bulge anteriorly, touching side of examiner's finger

FEMORAL

Least common hernia, more common in women than in men. Originates below inguinal ligament, more lateral than inguinal hernia. Never enters scrotum

ABNORMALITIES ON RECTAL EXAMINATION

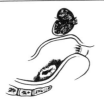

CANCER OF THE RECTUM. A firm to hard nodule or a rolled, irregular edge of an ulcerated cancer

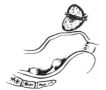

POLYP OF THE RECTUM. A soft mass that may or may not be on a stalk. May not be palpable

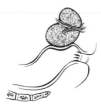

BENIGN PROSTATIC HYPERPLASIA. An enlarged, nontender, smooth, firm but slightly elastic prostate gland. Benign prostatic hyperplasia can cause symptoms without palpable enlargement.

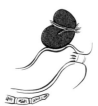

ACUTE PROSTATITIS. A prostate that is very tender, swollen, and firm because of acute infection

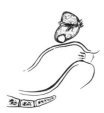

CANCER OF THE PROSTATE. A hard area in the prostate that may or may not feel nodular

ABNORMALITIES OF THE VULVA AND URETHRAL MEATUS

ULCERS OF THE VULVA

SYPHILITIC CHANCRE. Usually firm and painless, often but not necessarily single

GENITAL HERPES. Painful, shallow, on red bases; usually several or multiple

ULCERATED CARCINOMA OF THE VULVA. Most common in elderly women but not limited exclusively to them

RAISED LESIONS ON THE VULVA

EPIDERMOID CYST. Small, firm, round, smooth

VENEREAL WARTS (CONDYLOMATA ACUMINATA). Irregular in surface (warty), often multiple

SECONDARY SYPHILIS (CONDYLOMATA LATA). Slightly raised, flattened papules, round or oval, covered by a gray exudate

CARCINOMA OF THE VULVA. Raised, red, variable in appearance, may be ulcerated

BARTHOLIN'S GLAND INFECTION. A swelling in the posterior labium; tender and red when acute, cystic when chronic

RED SWELLINGS OF THE URETHRAL MEATUS

URETHRAL CARUNCLE. A small swelling on the posterior aspect of the urethral meatus

PROLAPSED URETHRAL MUCOSA. A ring of swollen red mucosa surrounding the urethral meatus

VAGINITIS

	Discharge	Other Symptoms
TRICHOMONAS **VAGINITIS**	Yellowish green, often profuse, may be malodorous	Itching, vaginal soreness, dyspareunia
CANDIDA **VAGINITIS**	White, curdy, often thick, not malodorous	Itching, vaginal soreness, external dysuria, dyspareunia
BACTERIAL VAGINOSIS	Gray or white, thin, homogeneous, scant, malodorous	Fishy genital odor
ATROPHIC VAGINITIS	Variable in color, consistency, and amount; may be blood tinged; rarely profuse	Itching, dysuria, dyspareunia

VAGINITIS

Vulva	Vagina	Laboratory Assessment
May be red	May be normal or red, with red spots, petechiae	Saline wet mount for trichomonads
Often red and swollen	Often red with white patches of discharge	KOH preparation for branching hyphae
Usually normal	Usually normal	Saline wet mount for "clue cells," "whiff test" with KOH for fishy odor
Atrophic	Atrophic, dry, pale; may be red, petechial, ecchymotic; possible erosions or adhesions	

RELAXATIONS OF THE PELVIC FLOOR

When the pelvic floor is weakened, various structures may become displaced. These displacements are seen best when the patient strains down.

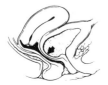

A **CYSTOCELE** is a bulge of the anterior wall of the upper part of the vagina, together with the urinary bladder above it.

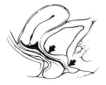

A **CYSTOURETHROCELE** involves both the bladder and the urethra as they bulge into the anterior vaginal wall throughout most of its extent.

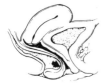

A **RECTOCELE** is a bulge of the posterior vaginal wall, together with a portion of the rectum.

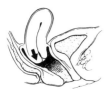

A **PROLAPSED UTERUS** has descended down the vaginal canal. There are three degrees of severity: first, still within the vagina (as illustrated); second, with the cervix at the introitus; and third, with the cervix outside the introitus.

COMMON VARIATIONS IN THE CERVIX

The **OS** may be round, oval, or slitlike.

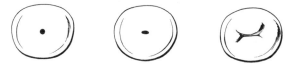

LACERATIONS from vaginal deliveries may be unilateral transverse, bilateral transverse, or stellate.

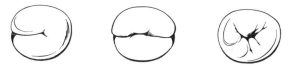

The **EPITHELIUM** of a normal cervix may be all squamous or both squamous and columnar. Retention (nabothian) cysts may be present.

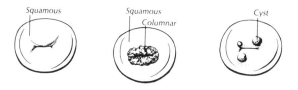

ABNORMALITIES OF THE CERVIX

CARCINOMA OF THE CERVIX. An irregular, hard mass suggests cancer. Early lesions cannot be detected by physical examination alone.

ENDOCERVICAL POLYP. A bright red, smooth mass that protrudes from the os suggests a polyp. It bleeds easily.

MUCOPURULENT CERVICITIS. A yellowish exudate emerging from the cervical os suggests this diagnosis. Causes include *Chlamydia* and gonococcal infections.

Columnar epithelium Vaginal adenosis
Collar

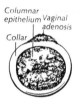

FETAL EXPOSURE TO DIETHYLSTILBESTROL. Several changes may be seen: a collar of tissue around the cervix, columnar epithelium that covers the cervix or extends to the vaginal wall (then termed *vaginal adenosis*), and, rarely, carcinoma of the vagina.

POSITIONS OF THE UTERUS AND UTERINE MYOMAS

An **ANTEVERTED UTERUS** lies in a forward position at roughly a right angle to the vagina. This is the most common position. *Anteflexion*—a forward flexion of the uterine body in relation to the cervix—often coexists.

A **RETROVERTED UTERUS** is tilted posteriorly with its cervix facing anteriorly.

A **RETROFLEXED UTERUS** has a posterior tilt that involves the uterine body but not the cervix. A uterus that is retroflexed or retroverted may be felt only through the rectal wall; some cannot be felt at all.

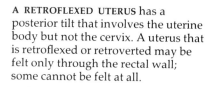

A **MYOMA OF THE UTERUS** is a very common, benign tumor that feels firm and often irregular. There may be more than one. A myoma on the posterior surface of the uterus may be mistaken for a retrodisplaced uterus; one on the anterior surface may be mistaken for an anteverted uterus.

THE DIAGNOSIS OF PREGNANCY

SUGGESTIVE SYMPTOMS IN FIRST TRIMESTER

No menstrual periods

Nausea with or without vomiting

Breast tenderness

Urinary frequency

Fatigue

PHYSICAL SIGNS —in weeks from the last menstrual period

6 TO 8 WEEKS

Softening of the uterine isthmus—the first clinical
manifestation of pregnancy (*Hegar's sign*)

Rounding of the body of the uterus into a globular shape

Softening of the cervix so that it feels like lips, not like the
nose

Purplish color of the vaginal and cervical mucosa

12 WEEKS

Fetal heart audible with Doptone

18 WEEKS

Fetal heart audible with fetoscope

24 WEEKS

Fetal movements usually palpable by examiner

12 TO 36 WEEKS

A rise in the fundal height:

To calculate *expected date of confinement* (*EDC*): Add 7 days
to the first day of last menstrual period, subtract 3 months,
and add 1 year.

CHRONIC VASCULAR INSUFFICIENCY

	Arterial	Deep Venous
PAIN	Intermittent claudication, possibly pain at rest	Aching on dependency
PULSES	Decreased or absent	Normal, but may be obscured by edema
COLOR	Pallor on elevation, rubor on dependency	Normal, or cyanotic on dependency. Pigmentation around the ankle
TEMPERATURE	Cool	Normal
EDEMA	Absent or mild	Present, often marked
SKIN CHANGES	Thin, shiny, atrophic; decreased hair; ridged, thickened nails	Brown pigment near the ankle, stasis dermatitis, and possible thickening of the skin with narrowing of the leg
ULCERS, IF ANY	Toes, points of trauma	At the sides of the ankle, especially medially
GANGRENE	May be present	Absent

PERIPHERAL CAUSES OF EDEMA

	Ortho-static Edema	Lymph-edema	Lip-edema	Deep Venous Insufficiency
EDEMA	Soft, pitting	Soft early, becomes hard and non-pitting	Minimal, if any	Soft, pitting; may become hard and nonpitting
SKIN THICKENING	Absent	Marked	Absent	Occasional
ULCERATION	Absent	Rare	Absent	Common
PIGMENTATION	Absent	Absent	Absent	Common
FOOT SWELLING	Yes	Yes	No	Yes
BILATERALITY	Always	Often	Always	Occasional

ABNORMALITIES OF THE HANDS

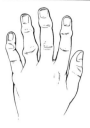

OSTEOARTHRITIS. Hard, dorsolateral nodules on the distal interphalangeal joints (*Herberden's nodes*) and, less commonly, similar nodules on the proximal interphalangeal joints (*Bouchard's nodes*)

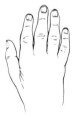

ACUTE RHEUMATOID ARTHRITIS. Tenderness, pain, stiffness, and swelling, affecting mainly the proximal interphalangeal and metacarpophalangeal joints

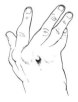

CHRONIC RHEUMATOID ARTHRITIS. Chronic swelling and thickening of the proximal interphalangeal and metacarpophalangeal joints; ulnar deviation of the fingers; muscular atrophy; rheumatoid nodules

Boutonniere (A) and *swan neck* (B) deformities may also be seen

(continued)

ABNORMALITIES OF THE HANDS
(Continued)

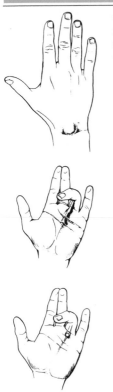

GANGLION. A cystic, round, usually nontender swelling along a tendon sheath or joint capsule. The wrist is a common site, but a ganglion may occur elsewhere.

DUPUYTREN'S CONTRACTURE. A thickening of the palmar fascia, first felt as a nodule near the distal palmar crease. A fibrotic cord then develops, and a flexion contraction involving the finger may ensue.

TRIGGER FINGER. A painless nodule in a flexor tendon of the palm, near the head of the metacarpal. Too big to slide easily into the tendon sheath on extension, it necessitates extra effort or force. A snap is felt and heard when it pops through.

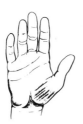

THENAR ATROPHY. Wasting of the muscles of the thenar eminence. It suggests a disorder of the median nerve.

SWOLLEN OR TENDER ELBOWS

Lateral epicondylitis

Arthritis

Olecranon bursitis

Rheumatoid nodules

EPICONDYLITIS	A painful, tender lateral epicondyle suggests *lateral epicondylitis* (tennis elbow). Extension of the wrist against resistance increases the pain.
	A painful, tender medial epicondyle (not illustrated) suggests *medial epicondylitis* (pitcher's, golfer's, or Little League elbow). Wrist flexion against resistance increases the pain.
ARTHRITIS	Tenderness and swelling in the groove between the olecranon process and the lateral epicondyle suggest arthritis of the elbow joint.
OLECRANON BURSITIS	Swelling superficial to the olecranon bursa suggests olecranon bursitis. It may be acute or chronic.
RHEUMATOID NODULES	Rheumatoid nodules are subcutaneous, firm, and nontender. They occur along the extensor surface of the ulna and may be attached to the underlying periosteum. They are associated with rheumatoid arthritis or acute rheumatic fever.

PAINFUL, TENDER SHOULDERS

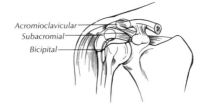

Acromioclavicular
Subacromial
Bicipital

SUBACROMIAL TENDERNESS

Tenderness in the subacromial area suggests either *rotator cuff tendinitis* (the impingement syndrome) or *calcific tendinitis*. The latter typically has a more acute onset and course.

TENDERNESS OVER THE BICEPS TENDON

Tenderness over the long head of the biceps tendon suggests *bicipital tendinitis*. With the patient's arm at the side and the elbow flexed to 90°, supination against resistance increases the pain.

ACROMIOCLAVICULAR JOINT TENDERNESS

Tenderness over the acromioclavicular joint (in the absence of recent injury that could also explain it) suggests acromioclavicular arthritis. Shrugging the shoulders often increases the pain, but movement limited to the glenohumeral joint does not.

ABNORMALITIES OF THE FEET

ACUTE GOUTY ARTHRITIS. A hot, red, painful, and tender swelling often involving the first metatarsophalangeal joint

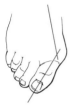

HALLUX VALGUS. A lateral deviation of the great toe in relation to the first metatarsal, which itself may be deviated medially. A bursa may form between the metatarsal head and the skin and become inflamed (a bunion).

HAMMER TOE. Hyperextension at the metatarsophalangeal joint with flexion at the proximal interphalangeal joint.

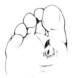

PLANTAR WART. A wart in the thick skin of the sole. It may be covered by a callus. Look for the small dark spots of a wart.

NEUROTROPHIC ULCER. A painless, often deep ulcer typically surrounded by callus. It occurs at pressure points in diabetic and other patients whose pain sensation is decreased or absent.

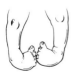

CLUBFOOT (TALIPES EQUINOVARUS). Characterized by forefoot adduction and by inversion and plantar flexion (equinus position) of the entire foot

SPINAL CURVATURES

NORMAL. A cervical concavity, a thoracic convexity, and a lumbar concavity

LORDOSIS. An accentuation of the normal lumbar concavity. It may accompany pregnancy, marked obesity, or kyphosis.

FLATTENING OF THE LUMBAR CURVE. Loss of the normal lumbar concavity. Causes include muscle spasm and ankylosing spondylitis.

LIST. A lateral tilt of the spine. A plumb line dropped from T1 falls lateral to the gluteal cleft. Muscle spasm associated with a herniated disc is a common cause.

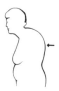

KYPHOSIS. An exaggerated, rounded thoracic convexity. It is common in aging, especially in women.

(continued)

SPINAL CURVATURES

GIBBUS. An angular, localized convexity due to one or more collapsed vertebrae. Causes include metastatic cancer and tuberculosis of the spine.

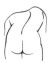

SCOLIOSIS. A lateral curvature of the spine. It is described by the location and direction of its chief convexity, here a thoracic scoliosis with convexity to the right. Compensating curves usually correct any list.

Forward flexion often makes scoliosis more evident.

FACIAL PARALYSIS

	Lesion of Peripheral Nervous System	Lesion of Central Nervous System
SIDE OF FACE AFFECTED	Same side as the lesion	Side opposite the lesion
LOWER FACE e.g., smiling, showing teeth	Weak or paralyzed	Weak or paralyzed
UPPER FACE, e.g., raising eyebrows, wrinkling forehead, closing eyes	Weak or paralyzed	Normal or slightly weak
COMMON CAUSE	Bell's palsy (injury to CN VII)	Cerebrovascular accident

GAIT AND POSTURE

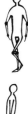

SPASTIC HEMIPARESIS. Arm held close to the side with joints flexed. Leg extended and foot plantar flexed. On walking, the toe scrapes or the leg is circumducted.

SCISSORS GAIT (BILATERAL SPASTIC PARESIS). A stiff gait in which the thighs cross forward on each other with each step. Steps are short.

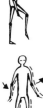

STEPPAGE GAIT (PERIPHERAL NERVE WEAKNESS). Because of foot drop, either dragging of the feet or lifting them high and slapping them down

SENSORY ATAXIA. Unsteady, wide-based gait, partially corrected by watching the ground. Feet thrown forward and outward and brought down on heels and then toes. Romberg test positive

CEREBELLAR ATAXIA. Unsteady, wide-based gait, with special difficulty on turns. In Romberg test, unsteadiness with eyes open or closed. Other cerebellar signs are associated.

PARKINSONISM. Stooped posture with flexed elbows and wrists. Slow, shuffling gait with short steps and stiff turns

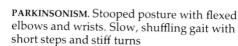

	Peripheral Nervous System Disorder	**Central Nervous System Disorder***
INVOLUNTARY MOVEMENTS	Often fasciculations	No fasciculations
MUSCLE BULK	Atrophy	Normal or mild atrophy (disuse)
MUSCLE TONE	Decreased or absent	Increased, spastic
MUSCLE STRENGTH	Decreased or lost	Decreased or lost
COORDINATION	Unimpaired, though limited by weakness	Slowed and limited by weakness
REFLEXES		
DEEP TENDON	Decreased or absent	Increased
PLANTAR	Flexor or absent	Extensor
ABDOMINALS	Absent	Absent

MOTOR

* *Upper motor neuron*

DISORDERS

Parkinsonism (Basal Ganglia Disorder)	Cerebellar Disorder
Resting tremors	Intention tremors
Normal	Normal
Increased, rigid	Decreased
Normal or slightly decreased	Normal or slightly decreased
Good, though slowed and often tremulous	Impaired, ataxic
Normal or decreased	Normal or decreased
Flexor	Flexor
Normal	Normal

INVOLUNTARY MOVEMENTS

TREMORS. Rhythmic oscillations that may be most evident (1) on movement (intention), (2) at rest, or (3) when maintaining a posture

INTENTION TREMORS

RESTING TREMORS

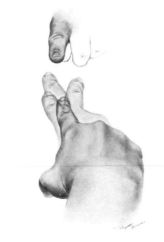

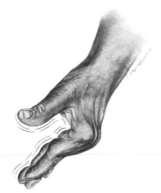

POSTURAL TREMORS

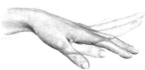

FASCICULATIONS. Fine, rapid flickering of muscle bundles

CHOREA. Brief, rapid, irregular, jerky; face, head, arms, or hands

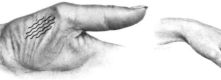

(continued)

INVOLUNTARY MOVEMENTS

ATHETOSIS. Slow, twisting, writhing; face, distal limbs

DYSTONIA. Grotesque, twisted postures, often in trunk or, as shown, in neck (*spasmodic torticollis*)

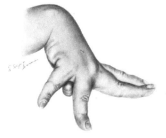

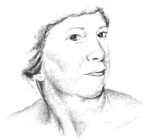

TICS. Brief, irregular, repetitive, coordinated movements, e.g., winking, shrugging

ORAL–FACIAL DYSKINESIAS. Rhythmic, repetitive, bizarre movements of face, mouth

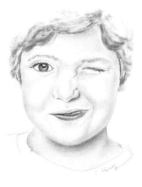

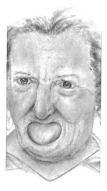

DERMATOMES

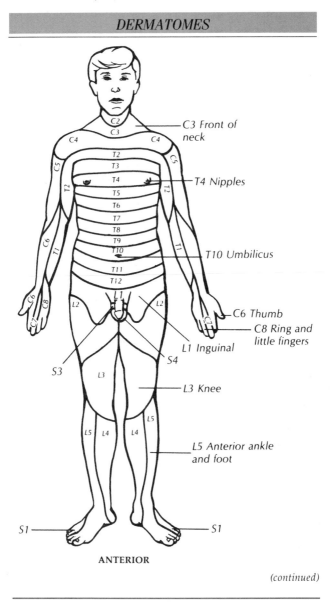

C3 Front of neck

T4 Nipples

T10 Umbilicus

C6 Thumb

C8 Ring and little fingers

L1 Inguinal

L3 Knee

L5 Anterior ankle and foot

ANTERIOR

(continued)

DERMATOMES

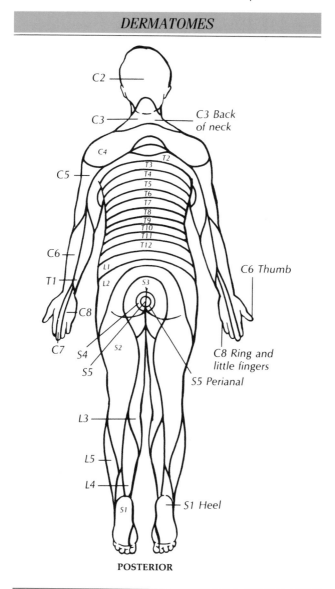

POSTERIOR

ABNORMAL POSTURES IN COMA

DECORTICATE RIGIDITY

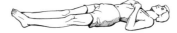

Occurs in lesions of corticospinal tracts in or near the cerebral hemispheres. When unilateral, this is the posture of chronic spastic hemiplegia.

DECEREBRATE RIGIDITY

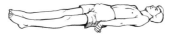

Occurs in severe metabolic coma or in structural coma involving the diencephalon, midbrain, or pons

FLACCID HEMIPLEGIA

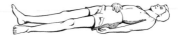

Occurs early in the course of unilateral lesions of the corticospinal tract

METABOLIC AND STRUCTURAL COMA

	Metabolic	Structural
RESPIRATORY PATTERN	If regular, normal or hyperventilation. If irregular, Cheyne–Stokes	Irregular, especially Cheyne–Stokes or ataxic breathing
PUPILS	Equal, reactive to light. (If pinpoint, use magnifier.) May be fixed, dilated from anticholinergics, hypothermia	Unequal or unreactive to light. Midposition and fixed in midbrain compression. Dilated and fixed in compression of cranial nerve III by herniation
LEVEL OF CONSCIOUSNESS	Changes after pupils change	Changes before pupils change
CAUSES INCLUDE:	Uremia, liver failure	Epidural, subdural, intracerebral hemorrhage
	Alcohol, drugs	Cerebral infarct or embolus
	Hypothyroidism	
	Anoxia, ischemia	Tumor, abscess
	Meningitis, encephalitis	Lesion in brainstem or cerebellum
	Hyper- or hypothermia	
	Hyper- or hypoglycemia	

ATTRIBUTES OF CLINICAL DATA

Validity—the closeness with which a measurement reflects the true value of an object

Reliability—the reproducibility of a measurement

Sensitivity, specificity, and *predictive values* are illustrated in a 2 × 2 table, as shown below in an example of 200 people, half of whom have the disease in question. A prevalence of 50% is much higher than is usually found in a clinical situation. Because the positive predictive value increases with prevalence, its calculated value here is accordingly and unrealistically high.

		Disease		
		Present	**Absent**	
+		**95** true positive observations *a*	**10** false positive observations *b*	**105** total positive observations
Observation				
−		**5** false negative observations *c*	**90** true negative observations *d*	**95** total negative observations
		100 total persons with the disease	**100** total persons without the disease	**200** total persons

$$\text{Sensitivity} = \frac{a}{a + c} = \frac{95}{95 + 5} \times 100 = 95\%$$

$$\text{Specificity} = \frac{d}{b + d} = \frac{90}{90 + 10} \times 100 = 90\%$$

$$\text{Positive predictive value} = \frac{a}{a + b} = \frac{95}{95 + 10} \times 100 = 90.5\%$$

$$\text{Negative predictive value} = \frac{d}{c + d} = \frac{90}{90 + 5} \times 100 = 94.7\%$$

CHAPTER 5

CLINICAL THINKING AND THE PATIENT'S RECORD

Bates, B. A POCKET GUIDE TO PHYSICAL EXAMINATION AND HISTORY TAKING, SECOND EDITION. © 1995 J.B. Lippincott Company.

Three parts of the patient's record are outlined in this chapter: (1) a comprehensive evaluation of an adult, from the history to the plan for the patient, (2) a problem list, and (3) a progress note. Clinical thinking is reviewed in the assessment portion of the comprehensive evaluation. Details of the history (see Chap. 1) are not repeated here. Major items in the physical examination are listed and should be expanded as indicated for a particular patient.

HISTORY

IDENTIFYING DATA, including name, address, age, place of birth, marital status, race, occupation, and religion

REFERRAL SOURCE, if any

SOURCE OF HISTORY

RELIABILITY, if relevant

CHIEF COMPLAINT(S)

PRESENT ILLNESS, including

A chronological account of the symptoms and their
    attributes
The meaning of the illness to the patient and his or her
    responses to it

PAST HISTORY

General health, as the patient perceives it
Childhood illnesses
Adult illnesses
Psychiatric illnesses
Injuries
Operations
Hospitalizations

CURRENT HEALTH STATUS

Current medications, prescribed or not
Allergies
Tobacco
Alcohol/drugs
Diet, including daily intake, restrictions, supplements
Screening tests
Immunizations
Sleep
Exercise/leisure
Environmental hazards
Safety measures

FAMILY HISTORY in diagrammatic or outline form. This should give the age and medical condition of at least the parents, siblings, spouse, and children, and the age at death, with its cause, of any who have died.

The symbols and structure of a family diagram are shown below.

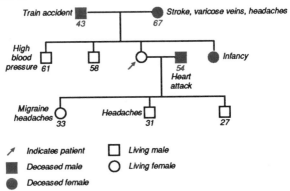

The family history should also include common familial or hereditary diseases and the presence of an illness similar to the patient's in any family member.

PSYCHOSOCIAL HISTORY

Home situation, significant others, and daily life
Important past experiences, such as school, work, marriage(s)
Outlook on the present and the future
Relevant religious beliefs

REVIEW OF SYSTEMS

General, including weight, weakness, fatigue, and fever
Skin
Head
Eyes
Ears
Nose and sinuses
Mouth and throat
Neck
Breasts
Respiratory
Cardiac
Gastrointestinal
Urinary
Genital
Peripheral vascular
Musculoskeletal
Neurologic
Hematologic
Endocrine
Psychiatric

PHYSICAL EXAMINATION

General survey, described in a succinct paragraph
Vital signs. Pulse rate, respiratory rate, blood pressure, and possibly temperature
Height and weight, in dressing gown if possible
Skin. Color, texture, lesions; hair and nails

Head. Hair, scalp, skull, face

Eyes. Vision, visual fields; conjunctiva, sclera; cornea, iris, lens; pupils (size, shape, reactions to light), extraocular movements; ophthalmoscopic examination

Ears. Auricles, canals, drums, auditory acuity, and, if indicated, Weber and Rinne tests

Nose. Mucosa, septum, sinus tenderness

Mouth. Lips, oral mucosa, gums, teeth, tongue, pharynx

Neck. Thyroid gland, trachea

Lymph nodes. Cervical, axillary, epitrochlear, inguinal

Thorax/lungs. Breathing (pattern, effort, sound), shape of chest, fremitus, percussion note, breath sounds, adventitious (added) sounds

Cardiovascular. Carotid pulses, jugular venous pressure, apical impulse, heart sounds, extra sounds, heart murmurs

Breasts. Size, symmetry, tenderness, masses

Abdomen. Shape, scars. Bowel sounds. Percussion note and pattern. Tenderness, including costovertebral angle tenderness; masses. Liver, spleen, kidneys, aorta

Genitalia
- Male. Penis, scrotum and contents, including testes; hernias
- Female. Vulva, vagina, cervix, uterus (size, shape, position), adnexa. Rectovaginal examination

Rectum. Anus, rectum, and (in men) prostate. Stool for occult blood

Peripheral vascular. Skin color, peripheral pulses, edema, varicose veins

Musculoskeletal. Deformities, swollen or tender joints. Back (curvatures or tenderness). Range of motion

Neurologic
- Cranial nerves (not already described)
- Motor system: body position, involuntary movements, muscle bulk, muscle tone, strength, coordination (rapid alternating movements, point-to-point movements)
- Gait and stance (Romberg test, pronator drift)
- Sensory system: pain, light touch, position, vibration, discriminative senses
- Reflexes

Mental status, in the detail indicated
- Appearance and behavior
- Speech and language
- Mood

- Thought and perception
- Memory and attention
- Higher cognitive functions

ASSESSMENT

For each problem identified from the patient's history, physical examination, or laboratory studies, summarize the relevant data and outline the clinical thinking that led to your formulation. The steps in the thought processes involved in this assessment are outlined below.

- Identify and list the abnormal findings in the data base, including symptoms, physical findings, and laboratory data.
- Cluster these findings into logical groups.
- Localize the findings anatomically as precisely as the data allow.
- Interpret the findings in terms of probable process.
- Make one or more hypotheses about the nature of the patient's problems.
- Eliminate hypotheses that do not explain the key findings or that are incompatible with them.
- Weigh the probability of competing hypotheses according to
  Their match with the findings
  Their probability in this particular patient (of the given age, sex, habits, geographic location, and other variables)
- Consider carefully the possibility of potentially life-threatening or treatable conditions even if they are less common and thus less likely.
- Establish a working definition of the problem(s) at the highest level of certainty and explicitness that the data allow.
- Recall that various findings can be evaluated according to their validity, reliability, sensitivity, specificity, and predictive values. Definitions of these terms are given on p. 208.

PLAN

For each problem, develop a plan in three categories:

- Diagnostic
- Therapeutic
- Educational

PROBLEM LIST

This is a numbered list of problems that is usually placed in the front of the patient's chart. The name of a problem (but not its number) is modified if additional data change the assessment. In the following example, the clinician crossed out "Edema, left leg" after making the new, more precise diagnosis of deep venous thrombosis.

Date problem entered	No.	Active problems	Inactive problems
9-24-94	1.	~~Edema, left leg~~	
9-25-94	1.	Deep venous thrombosis, left iliofemoral vein	
9-25-94	2.	Acute chest pain and dyspnea	.

PROGRESS NOTE

Include the date and perhaps the time. Give the number and name of the problem, followed by

- S. (Subjective) The patient's report
- O. (Objective) The clinician's observations
- A. (Assessment) The clinician's interpretation of what is going on
- P. (Plan) Further plans, diagnostic, therapeutic, or educational

INDEX